I Am Someone You Know

The Fight for Recovery and Mental Health

© 2025 David Shamszad

All rights reserved. No portion of this book may be reproduced, stored in a retrieval system, or transmitted in any form by any means – electronic, mechanical, photocopy, recording, scanning, or other – except for brief quotations in critical reviews or articles without the prior written permission of the publisher.

ISBN 979-8-9905562-5-6

Published in Phoenix, Arizona by Emissary Publishing.
Photography and Cover Artwork by Gabriel Berent

The views expressed by the author are those of the author and do not necessarily reflect the views of the publisher.

For Reza. Always be you.

Table of Contents

Prologue

Part One 1
    No Pulp
    Tower Records
    Gregarious
    Smacked Down

Part Two 22
    Six Foot Nothin'
    Sing the Body Electric
    Ham & Eggs
    Lehman, Bro
    Eight Bit

Part Three 40
    Kumbaya
    Juan
    Five Foot Nothin'
    Brandon
    Coffee Break

Part Four 62
    I
    II
    It Had a Name

    Justine
    Don't Operate Heavy Machinery

Part Five 81
    California Love
    The Doctor Will See You Now
    Hat Trick
    Goodnight, Sweet Prince
    No Balls, No Babies

Part Six 100
    Season's Greetings
    Come Out and Play
    III
    A Permanent Stain

Part Seven 122
    La Farmacia
    Don't Turn Off the Lights
    III
    We Need to Talk

Part Eight 143
    Paula
    Moderation
    Six Drinks and Six Strings

Part Nine 159
    New Balance
    Yes, Your Honor
    My Grandfather's Blood

Part Ten 178
    The Whale
    Doritos, Hot Pockets, and Vicodin
    Two Steps Back
    Always Faithful
    V
    VI
    VII

Part Eleven 210
    The Quail
    II
    Ringing in the New Year
    IV
    V
    Bcc:

Part Twelve 231
    Before the Dawn
    Midnight Basketball
    Tiki Torches
    A Group of One
    The Doctor Will See You, Again
    A Family Crest
    I Am Someone You Know

Epilogue 251

Prologue

White walls. White bed sheets. White plastic bracelet on my wrist... Psychiatric Hospital. *No, this can't be real. Please be a dream.*

Last thing I remember is the knife. I can still see it. The old blade stretching the skin. Pressing harder. Then... here.

Annie. She's going to think I'm insane. Maybe I am.

Work. There's no one to cover me. I should be there doing my job. I should—

"Hi, there. Good to see you again. How are you feeling today?"

"Oh, um, okay. Wait, have we talked before?"

"Yes, we spoke yesterday when you arrived. I'm sure you must feel very disoriented."

"A little. I don't know."

"Are the medications we gave you having any side-effects that you are experiencing?"

"I can't tell if I'm awake or not."

"I understand. Why don't we start by just talking about what you've been going through as of late?"

"I haven't really slept for a couple of weeks. Only if I'm drunk. I feel like... so much joy some of the time. Like a fucking dream. But then... a nightmare. Violent, twisted thoughts racing through my mind. And it all feels so real." *I never talk about any of this. But I don't care right now. Maybe it's the pills.*

"Continue, if you can."

"And lately I've wanted to hurt myself. I think about jumping in front of cars or throwing myself off a bridge. I drink to make it go away. To sleep."

"And… " *Why am I telling him all of this—I should stop. But what's the difference?*

"Yesterday—fuck, man. Yesterday, I tried to cut my wrists open because I thought the pain would leave if I did."

"You mentioned drinking. How often are you using alcohol?"

Don't go there. "I think I need to lie down. I don't want to be awake anymore."

What is happening to me? I knew something was wrong. Years ago, I knew. I ran from it. Ran, ran, ran. But it finally got me. And now there's… so much fucking pain.

Annie. Imagining you are here. My chin and lips sinking into the soft space between your neck and shoulder. I could die now and make this moment with you the last I ever have.

Part One

Chapter 1 - No Pulp

I stood in the doorway of the second-grade classroom while twenty pairs of little eyeballs fixated on me. I was new, didn't know a soul, and I had a big hearing aid draped over my left ear. I hated having to explain what it was to these unfamiliar kids. Before the teacher could come help me find my way, a cheery blond boy skipped over to me.

"I'm Peter! Use this cubby. It's not anybody's. And you can sharpen your pencils over here."

That was new to me. We didn't have our own pencils at my first school. Teachers just gave them out when we needed them and snatched them back when we were done. After I started my fourth pencil, I heard some cackling.

Peter leaned into my ear and said, "You don't have to do the whole box all at once. Just do some more when you run out." He was my first friend. And after he shoved some kid who made fun of my hearing aid, he became my best friend.

I'd have my first cigarette with Peter—an American Spirit. I'd get high for the first time with Peter—out of a soda can. And I'd get drunk for the first time with Peter, too—a fifth of Smirnoff.

Over the summer break, before freshman year, my parents left town for a weekend. My two sisters and I were supposed to spend the night with friends. Peter and I planned to get some alcohol, stay at my house alone, and drink it—nothing else. We'd drunk before, but just a few sips here and there. Enough to feel our cheeks flush with warm blood and a tingle in our arms and chests. But we wanted to know what came next. We wanted to get fucked up.

My dad's stuff was out of the question. He had a full liquor cabinet of bottles in all different colors, shapes, and sizes. Once, we took a few small sips of tequila from a small bottle at the back of the highest shelf, just to see what it tasted like and how much it burned when it touched our tongues. I thought my dad couldn't possibly notice... but he did. And it sure as shit wasn't gonna happen again.

We decided to walk a mile to the grocery store and find a grown-up willing to help. After a half dozen flatly rejected us, I suggested, "Maybe we should just try to get some weed instead, dude."

But before we used our twenty bucks for some shitty marijuana, we found our hero. He was tall and slender, with scruffy hair brushing his shoulders, a cool leather jacket, and ripped jeans. He reminded me of John Bender from *The Breakfast Club*. Just by his looks, I was sure—he was our guy.

"Hey, man, do you think you could get us something to drink?" I tried to sound relaxed, like I'd done it before.

He stared at me for a few long seconds. I couldn't tell if he was deciding whether to help us out or to laugh in my face.

"Alright, boys. What do you want?"

"A fifth of Smirnoff," I said. We knew the sub-premium vodka brand would fit in our scant budget and leave us with enough left over for something to chase it. And maybe some extra cigarettes.

When he came out of the store, he handed me the vodka in a brown paper bag. I waited for him to pass me the seven remaining dollars.

"Ummm… Can we get the change?"

He stared at me for a few more long seconds until we scrammed, seven dollars poorer than expected. We'd have to make due without a chaser, but, fortunately, Pete had enough blue American Spirits for the night.

We didn't have any particular plan for the night. No parties, no drinking games—nothing but drinking as much as we could and seeing what happened. We felt like eager explorers embarking on a new, long-awaited adventure. The night could have been perfect.

But then the phone rang.

"Hello?"

"Hey, Dave! What are you up to?"

When I was in eighth grade and Caitlin was a freshman, she and I made out a few times. She had a big crush on me after that, but I didn't feel the same way. I felt guilty and did not want to lead her on, so I told her I just wanted to be friends. But it never wholly deterred her.

"Hey, what's up? Uh, nothing really. Pete is here. We're just hanging out by ourselves tonight," I answered.

"Can I come?"

"Well," I paused, trying to come up with an answer. "My parents are gone, and I'm not allowed to have anyone over."

"But you already have someone over."

Whoops. "Yeah, but, I mean, we aren't really doing much. Prolly just gonna watch a movie or something." *Good lie.*

"That sounds great, actually. Let me join you guys!"

Shit. "Whatever, okay. That's cool, I guess." *Should have let it go to voicemail.*

Caitlin had started hooking up with a guy named Damon. He was older than us and had been expelled from school for fighting. I was sure he wouldn't love the idea of Caitlin coming over to drink with us. When she got there a couple hours later, she reached into her bag and pulled out a bottle of white wine.

"We already have some stuff," I said. "I don't think we need more."

"Well, I like wine better anyway. More for me!"

We laid our bounty out on the counter. Three glasses, the cheap vodka, and the cheaper wine. Even though we had just two bottles and a trio of cups, we spread them apart to make it seem like we had a full wet bar. None of us knew how much we needed to drink to get *drunk*, so we just started drinking and figured we would know when to stop. Holy moly, did the first swig of vodka burn.

"Ha!" Caitlin laughed when she saw my face recoil. "You didn't get anything to chase it with? What about some of that orange juice?" She'd seen it in the fridge.

"No way. Don't touch that," Peter said. He knew from prior forays into our fridge that my dad's precious, pulpy, fresh-squeezed Odwalla was as off-limits as the liquor. Despite the harshness of the vodka to our untrained palates, it wasn't worth going near the OJ. "It has the pulp anyway… gross."

"Do you feel anything yet?" Peter asked the group.

"I'm definitely starting to get a little drunk!" Caitlin chirped.

"Yeah, it's kicking in, for sure," I understated.

From there, it didn't take long. Minutes later, we were slurring our words and barely upright. Mission accomplished—we'd gotten definitively fucked up. We went outside and crashed onto some lawn chairs. Every joke we told was hilarious. Every sensation we felt in our hands and faces was blissful. Caitlin stood up and twirled around playfully, letting her arms extend outward, smiling up at the night sky. Soon enough, the whole fifth *and* Caitlin's wine had disappeared.

But then—before any of us knew it—everything changed. The house began to spin. It got hard to talk. Hard to even think. The fun wore off. I laid down on the floor of the kitchen, dizzy, disoriented, and growing nauseous.

Suddenly, Caitlin was on top of me, trying to kiss me.

"What are you doing? Come on, stop it." I tried to laugh it off.

Even in my current state, I knew it wasn't a good idea. We were just friends—plus she had a big, fairly scary boyfriend. I stumbled to the living room couch. If I closed my eyes, I thought, maybe I could just fall asleep. It worked, until I woke up to Caitlin on top of me again. This time, she kissed me more aggressively, and she had no shirt on. Her skin pressed into mine, bare and warm. I'd never felt a girl's breasts like that. Never had them on my face or in my mouth. She took my hand and slid it down… there. I'd never done that either. I wanted to, but not like this.

"No, stop. We have to go to bed."

I already felt nauseous, but that encounter tipped me over the edge. I buried my head in the toilet and emptied out my insides.

Chapter 2 - Tower Records

Still drunk when we woke up, we all did our haphazard best to clean up the house, scouring for any and all evidence of the night before. Caitlin and I shared an awkward, clunky hug with our asses sticking out.

That night at home, I bullshitted my way through dinner with my parents, telling them about bike rides we didn't take and movies we didn't watch. I'd hoped for a massive rush of relief when I finally got to my bedroom, but I had no such reprieve. Guilt washed over me, like none I'd felt before, after having broken just about every rule my parents had.

Right on cue, my mom hurled open my bedroom door, smacking it into the wall. She stared at me for several long seconds with an expression I'd never seen before.

"What the hell is this?" She demanded, while a bra hung from one finger.

Oh, fuck. We'd cleaned up the bottles, glasses, and cigarette butts we'd accumulated. But Caitlin had forgotten one crucial item.

Seconds later, I could feel the vibration of my dad's deep, angry bellow echoing through the house. "Every time they get together, we get fucked over!"

"Just let me talk to David and find out what's going on."

Please, convince him to stay away from me.

"Fine. You talk to the little shit," he said, using his go-to designation for me when I was in trouble.

"You'd better tell me everything," she warned, still standing in the doorway. "Was there alcohol?"

"Pete and Caitlin came over, and we got some vodka," I said. Knowing what her next question would be, I added, "Some random guy bought it for us."

"How much did you drink?" she asked.

"Not a lot. A couple of those small, flat bottles." My first lie.

"And you finished it all?"

"No." Second lie.

"Did anyone have sex?"

"What? No, of course not." That was true, at least.

Mom heard him coming before I did. She pulled back into the hallway outside my door. "I said I would talk to him. Please let me handle—" But he rocketed past right past her.

At the foot of my bed, atop a short bookshelf, sat my prized Sony stereo system—dual cassette decks, compact disc player, two detachable speakers, the works—along with a few huge stacks of CDs arranged in alphabetical order. I'd given Tower Records just about every dollar I'd collected from chores and summer jobs. If only it had been enough.

My dad tore down the CD towers in one swipe. Plastic cases flew through the air and exploded against the wall behind me. Wu Tang Clan, Dr. Dre, and Notorious B.I.G all laid in pieces. He pushed my head back into the corner with his index finger.

"Why? Why do you want to hurt us?"

I looked away—his stare was too scary. I thought if I avoided eye contact, it might let the anger flow through him faster. *Let him see your fear, weakness, and guilt.*

They grounded me for six months. School and back every day—that was it. Weekends were virtual house arrest. But I felt relieved. I deserved it. The hardest part of staying home all the time, though, was seeing my parents so much. I could feel their searing pain and anger every time they glanced in my direction.

School, at least, got me out of the house and took my mind off Peter, Caitlin, and my ripshit mad parents. I went to a new school across the Bay, and no one knew me. I could forget about the trouble I had gotten in and just let the teachers' monotones distract me.

A few weeks into my punishment, while I sat upstairs in my room trying to unravel some impossible algebra homework, I heard a thunderous knock on the front door, followed by a deep, angry voice.

"Where the fuck is David?"

I crept towards the open window. *Damon*. He was sixteen, but he looked like a grown-ass man. *Fuck me. This can't be real. He's going to kick my ass.*

"What's going on, dude?" *Playing dumb ain't gonna work.*

"You know what I'm doing here! You hooked up with my girl! Get the fuck outside!"

Oh, man, she told him? I guess I would, too.

"Sorry, man. But I promise not much happened." I wasn't about to try to explain that I'd tried to stop her advances.

"Come down here." His volume lowered. "I just want to talk and get this figured out."

Figured out? I wasn't buying that.

"My parents are going to be home any minute. Just leave," I pleaded, "and I promise I'll call you tomorrow."

The next day, he showed up at Peter's school and scoured the hallways looking for him before getting escorted out. He never tracked down Peter. And I never called him back. But word spread quickly of his visits, leaving peers and parents wondering what kind of boys Peter and I were. Bad ones, I was sure.

Over and over again, I asked myself how I could have let all of this all happen. But even after weighing my guilt, my parents' anger, and all my smashed CDs, I knew I was no less enthralled with alcohol, even if its reciprocation felt a bit cruel. I loved the tingling anticipation while we waited for Bender from *The Breakfast Club* to come out of the store. I loved the burning sensation as it touched my tongue, throat, and stomach. I loved the feeling of freedom I found in being hopelessly intoxicated.

But that love scared me. I knew it would only get me into more trouble. And so I decided I'd be better off staying away.

For the rest of freshman year, I kept to myself. I felt anxious, insecure, and distracted. Classes at my new school were already fucking hard to begin with. I'd gone to a struggling, public middle school in Oakland where classes erupted into chaos half the time. When I got to a small, private high school, the academics hit me like a blizzard.

I fell behind so quickly. After my first semester, I'd already notched two Fs. It didn't help that I'd long since ditched my hearing aid after getting peppered with enough "Deafy Duck" jabs. I started smoking weed to blot out my embarrassment and discomfort. I got high after school before getting on the bus or late at night on midnight strolls around the block. I didn't even love getting high. It just took me somewhere *else* for a few hours.

By the end of freshman year, my GPA had fallen below a C average. The dean said I needed to go to summer school to make up credits for the classes I failed. And that wasn't all—if I didn't improve significantly when the fall semester came around, I'd be gone. I overheard my parents talking that night, debating whether it was even worth the headache or the tuition. *I'm nothing but a fuck-up.*

At Oakland High's summer session, I knew a few familiar faces from my middle school, including a giant of a teenager from East Oakland who, in the first week of sixth grade, stole my Discman—and *The Chronic,* still spinning inside when he snatched it out of my hand. I knew my parents were embarrassed that their son had to go to summer school. It was a long couple of months, and I was wrought with guilt.

Guilt had closely followed me my whole life. I felt guilty when my sisters were sad, as if I had the power to take their sadness and swallow it up. I felt guilty when our sixteen-year-old dog died, as if I failed to do something to make him live just a little longer. But *nothing* triggered guilt like my parents' disappointment.

Chapter 3 - Gregarious

My dad left Iran, alone, at the age of sixteen. He was estranged from his father, who, in turn, had been estranged from his own. Pain and abuse had plagued his family's legacy. He departed his home in Tehran as soon as he figured out how. He took with him only his soccer kit and a camera. He rode his incredible soccer talent around the world, first playing for a university in Germany and eventually landing at UC Berkeley, where he met my mom.

New to town, she'd just taken a gig making sandwiches at a local cafe. When she got to work on her first day, she found the whole staff protesting outside. With signs in hand, they shouted demands for better hours, better pay, better... everything. Before long, the young man who'd started the ad hoc strike strutted inside with his cohort behind him and told the owner he was ready to negotiate. The two of them went into the back while my mom and her new colleagues waited anxiously in the dining room.

"We have a deal!" announced my dad, to the cheers of grateful cooks and waiters.

My mom was smitten and came to fall in love with the handsome, confident, and persuasive young man. As good as my dad was as a soccer player and a deli-labor negotiator, he was even better with a camera. After college, with a bit of money saved up from working at the restaurant, he opened a small photo studio. By the time my older sister was born, he'd become one of the best photographers in the area.

Soon, he opened a bigger studio and began printing ads for all kinds of products. The brick masonry walls of his studio were adorned with glamorous prints he had done for clients—black backdrops with glossy close-ups of mascara-laden eyelashes, five-star plates from the hottest restaurants, or, in an uncanny twist, a pristine bottle of premium liquor.

He loved my mom, my sisters, and me, and he worked damn hard to provide us a comfortable life. But the love in his heart competed for space with unreconciled trauma from his past. He had left his home behind, but he couldn't leave the pain. Seeds of his old household were planted in our new one. Before I could remember, he'd found that alcohol gave him an illusory respite from the anguish he still held inside of him. But that deal with the devil poisoned him and, in turn, our home.

Despite all of my fear and anger, I loved him dearly. I knew he was much more than the pain he projected. He was the loving son who stared at a flickering candle and wept for hours after his estranged father passed away. He was the dependable parent who stayed up until three a.m. to help me finish a science project I'd put off until the last minute. He was the steadfast provider who worked tirelessly to make sure we had things he never did. He could shine bright like the sun, but he was so often trapped behind the darkest of clouds.

Each night, after work, he poured himself a regular drinking glass of tequila or whiskey. No ice. It seemed like he needed it before he could engage with us. He continued with beer or wine throughout dinner and the rest of the evening. On weekends, he always had a drink in his hand. We didn't go out much as a family. But if we did, he sometimes drove us there with one hand on the wheel and the other holding a glass of wine. Until I reached my early teens, I thought all grown-ups drank like he did.

My fifteenth birthday fell on a Sunday. Usually, we spent birthdays with family, but some kids from my new school proposed a little barbecue at the park to celebrate. I'd only just started making friends after returning for sophomore year, and I didn't want to decline.

"Is it okay if I go meet up with some friends? We were thinking of having a barbeque." As usual, I added, "No alcohol."

"You don't want to celebrate with your family?" my mom asked. It was only sort of a question.

"Well, it's not that I don't want to, I just thought this year I would do something with friends. But never mind, I can stay in if you—"

"No, go on. What do we care?" my dad jutted in.

The sky was overcast at the park, and drizzle spattered us throughout the day—not enough to call it off, but enough to put a damper on the mood. When I got home, my parents sat at the kitchen table eating dinner alone. My sisters had already gone upstairs to do homework. Without looking up, my dad took a sip of his drink and then said, "Hope you had fun with your friends."

I felt tired and dejected. My birthday was supposed to be fun. But the weather was shitty outside, and I felt a similar shittiness inside. "I'm sorry if I'm just a little bit more gregarious than you guys."

Gregarious. An admittedly superfluous word I'd picked up in class. He interpreted it as a slight. He wasn't wrong—I had meant it to sting a little bit.

My dad felt insecure about his English. So, when I started learning crafty SAT words like *gregarious,* he thought I used them to show him up. On very rare occasions, like this one, I did.

My dad sprang out of his seat. His soccer speed hadn't yet betrayed him. He darted around the island counter as I ran toward the stairs going to my room. I planned to shut the door and press my back against it, like I'd done many times before. But I never made it.

He grabbed my shoulders and pinned me against the kitchen cabinets. With one hand, he gripped my shirt collar. With the other, he grabbed the biggest knife in the wooden block and lodged it right between us. The butt of the handle pressed into my chest. The tip of the blade pressed into his.

"Is this what you want?" He pulled me in even harder, daring the knife to pierce his skin. "Would this make you happy?" he shouted.

I couldn't move or speak. I was afraid that if I tried to wrestle away, the knife would cut into him. I craned my head up towards the ceiling so I couldn't see it. *This can't be fucking real, can it?* I squeezed my eyes shut and waited. The moment he backed away, I sprinted to my room and slammed the door shut. I collapsed in a heap on the floor and wrapped my arms around my knees.

This is my fault, I thought. *Why did I go out all weekend? I should have known better. Why the fuck did I say "gregarious"? Who even says that stupid fucking word?!*

Not long after that, my mom asked him to leave. She'd endured too much, and she knew we'd endured enough, too. She told him he couldn't come back until he got sober. I felt so proud of her for summoning that courage. We didn't know if he would come back or, if he did, if anything would change. But he *did* come back. And, in time, things *were* different.

He never drank again, using the same courage that propelled him out on his own into the world at age sixteen. He pushed himself through years of therapy, AA meetings, and a daily hundred-and-five-degree yoga class. He wore a silver necklace with a pendant in the shape of a phoenix. Donning it every day reminded him that he'd started a new life.

It was better at home. We could see his efforts at restraint and patience. There were signs of hope, for the first time. Sadly, though, I had trouble forgiving the past. I loved him, and I felt grateful he had worked so hard to provide for me and my sisters. But I couldn't easily absolve him for the hurt he'd caused.

In the end, I would stay angry and estranged for as many years as I'd been subjected to the pain, if not more. Before I could acquire any empathy, I'd walk his line myself and let trauma seep from one generation to the next.

Chapter 4 - Smacked Down

I started studying harder in school. At first, I just wanted to make my parents proud of me—and to not go back to Oakland High. I still didn't wear my hearing aid, but I *did* sit in the front of the class so I could hear every word possible. Then, what started as self-preservation turned into something else. I became interested—curious, even—in what I learned. Mrs. Huntington had us read *Henry IV.* After I made some sense of the Elizabethan-era iambic pentameter, I realized Prince Hal and I could relate. He wasn't the only disappointment of a person perched on the verge of breaking because foul and ugly circumstances threatened to strangle him.

By the beginning of my junior year, a fire had lit under me. I loved all the subjects—reading, writing, and even chemistry. I didn't get in trouble anymore. Instead, I immersed myself in homework. I stopped getting high—I knew it would upset the magic I'd harnessed. I didn't even *want* to drink or smoke, realizing for the first time that success made me feel better than weed and alcohol ever did. The feelings I'd run away from—shame of who I was and the guilt of what I'd done—slowly became replaced by pride in my accomplishments.

I began doing more, finding new ways to earn respect at school and affection at home. Early in the morning before class, a couple days a week, a friend and I picked up day-old, unused food from restaurants and dropped it off at local homeless shelters. On occasional Saturdays, I volunteered at the soup kitchen to serve food to those in need. Even just a year prior, I wouldn't have ever imagined being the kind of person who did this.

I'd always been okay at sports, but I'd never stuck with anything long enough—or tried hard enough—to get very good. I decided to join the basketball squad and actually commit. Midway through our first suicides drill, I had to sprint to the garbage can instead of the baseline. After I came up for air and wiped some lingering puke from my face, I actually found myself invigorated. I'd never pushed my body that hard. My chest burned, but it was a good fire. My limbs felt dead, but it was a gratifying numbness. I stuck with basketball, despite the team having plenty of better shooters, rebounders, defenders, and passers. I gave it my all, and I stayed a consummate teammate and cheerleader.

As part of an AP history course, we took a week-long trip to the Southern states. My great-great-great-grandfather served as a general in the Civil War. I found a bust in his memory in Richmond, Virginia. A couple of generations later, my grandfather, Russell, became a brigadier general in the Marines and fought in World War II.

As a kid, I liked to wander around my grandfather's study like it was a museum. I'd run my hands over medals, plaques, and artifacts. I fixated on rows and rows of books about generals, wars, presidents, and politics. I gazed through the glass of his foreboding gun case, which housed a set of rifles perched on green felt racks. Gazed only—I was not allowed to lay a finger on it.

My grandfather was a high-achiever all his life. As far as I knew, he didn't get in trouble drinking or fuck around in school, like I had. I felt glad that he had lived to finally see me turn the corner. Over Christmas dinner, during junior year, he commended me.

"So, David, your mother tells me you've been doing a good job in school this year."

"Oh, yes. I've been trying to do better." I was taken aback. He didn't dole out praise often.

"Sounds like you've been doing more than just 'better.' Straight A's?"

"Um, yes. So far, at least."

"Well, keep it that way. What about the SAT?"

"I got fifteen-hundred."

"Is that good?"

"Yeah, it is, I guess."

"Where are you going to study?"

"I don't know, yet. Still waiting to hear back from Dartmouth."

"Well, if you don't get in, there's always the Marines."

"Who's ready for dessert?" *Thanks, Mom.*

During my senior year, WWE's *Thursday Night Smackdown* came to town. The Rock would be there. Stone Cold Steve Austin, Triple H, and the Undertaker, too. I'd wanted to see wrestling in person since I was a young kid watching the epic battles between the Ultimate Warrior and Hulk Hogan. On our way to the event, my mom called.

"David," she said, in a tone that made me nervous. *What did she find in my room this time?*

"Yeah? Is everything okay?"

"You got in."

I had pretty much written off getting into Dartmouth. It seemed almost as much of a long shot as the Rock inviting us backstage after *Smackdown*.

"What? No way. Are you sure? It's a big envelope?"

"Yes, a very big envelope. David, we're so proud of you."

By now, my friends were all looking at me. "Go have fun. We're so happy for you. See you later, honey."

"Guys—holy fucking shit. I got into Dartmouth."

"What?" said Brian, who was driving. "How the fuck did you pull that off?"

The imposter in me stood ready to answer. "Ha, no kidding. Lucky, I guess."

While the rest of the car gave me a chorus of congrats and light punches to my shoulders and chest, I sank into relief. I felt vindicated, having come a long way since almost getting kicked out of two schools.

When we pulled into the parking lot, someone got out some alcohol and cigarettes: a couple pints of Bacardi Limon—teenagers like that flavored shit—and a pack of Parliament Lights. The Capri Sun-flavored rum made its way around the circle. In a few beats, I'd have a decision to make. With the clear bottle of tangy rum dangled in front of me, someone shouted, "Come on, you only get into college once. And it's fucking *Smackdown,* dude!"

I guess that's true. I'll just have a little bit. I took one swig. But then, after the bottle made another full circle around the group, I took another. And then a couple more. Until it emptied. Sadly, the Rock lost to Triple H, who hit him with a chair when the ref had looked away. We lamented the Rock's fake coma with exaggerated cries and screams. I even ripped my Rock t-shirt in protest of Vince McMahon's treacherous storyline. We had a good day, and I didn't feel guilty for drinking. In fact, I even stumbled onto an idea: maybe—just maybe—my bad luck with alcohol was in the past.

With APs, college admissions, and SATs behind me, I tested my theory and started drinking more. Every other weekend, at first. Then, every Saturday. It didn't take long before I drank every Friday after school through the Saturday wee hours. And not only did I drink regularly, but I also got very, very fucked up, foraying into that dark, barely conscious territory—that mischief I swore I would leave behind sought me out again.

One night, I got into a fight with a security guard after a party got broken up. He doused my eyes with pepper spray and cracked me in the head with a MagLite. Both hurt, but the pepper spray burned worse. Friends poured a gallon of milk all over my head because one of them had heard it would help. It did not.

Soon after, a girl I'd slept with came up to me at a party and let me know she needed to tell me something in private. My heart rate tripled as we walked to an empty room in the house. *Pregnant? A boyfriend that wants to kill me?*

"I wanted to give you a heads-up that I have something."

"What do you mean you 'have something'?"

"Shhh. Don't be so loud," she said.

"Well, just tell me already. I'm super nervous right now."

"Chlamydia."

"Fuck," I said, though I was relieved we were talking about an STI and not a baby.

"It's not a huge deal. It goes away. There's pills."

"Well, do you have any?"

"What? On me? No, gross, dude. Just go to the doctor."

She didn't have to ask me to keep quiet about it. It would indeed stay *our* secret. And so I learned that Chlamydia doesn't burn as much as pepper spray, but it lasts much longer.

I finished the school year and the summer with more antics. Binge drinking. Drugs. Unprotected sex. Drunk driving. Along with my eyes from the pepper spray and my junk from the clap, the other thing burning was that familiar shame. The same one I'd felt after my mom found Caitlin's bra. I'd fought hard to become someone new that both my parents and I could be proud of.

But I'd let my guard down. The new person I had become—the one going to an Ivy League school and delivering food to soup kitchens—could disappear so quickly. *When I get to college, I'm gonna stay away from drinking. For real this time. And no fucking fraternities.*

Part Two

Chapter 1 - Six Foot Nothin'

The bus from the airport dropped me right in front of the huge quad in front of Dartmouth Hall. Eager kids darted back and forth across the town square made of neatly kept grass and intersecting paths. They moved at fast-forward speed—excited, like they knew where they were going and were eager to get there. I was an incoming freshman from California with wide eyes and not nearly enough winter clothes for college in New Hampshire.

Collections of brick buildings surrounded the quad, adorned with white columns and intricate moldings. Red, orange, and yellow trees painted the backdrop of this idyllic, picturesque, New England landscape, with an historic college at its center. I'd arrived at a special place. I had a picture of what my life would look like when I got to college—an archetype of a renaissance student, or something like that. I figured it included things like sitting in a circle on the quad and talking about the Classics, trying my hand at a lab course or two, and joining some clubs. And, I hoped, making the rugby or crew team. That seemed like an Ivy League sort of thing to do. I'd come to love the daily routine of high school basketball practice and the exhilaration of that last painful, self-questioning baseline-to-baseline sprint. Sadly, though, the recruiters for the basketball team must have lost my phone number.

During orientation week, a couple of big dudes on the quad sported their varsity rowing jackets—green and white with a cool "D" insignia. Each of them had a twelve-foot oar standing by their side.

Based on the little I'd gathered, it seemed like height was a key criterion for rowing. I sauntered over to them with my chin jilted up, trying to make myself appear taller—and more confident—than I really was.

Act cool. "Hey, fellas."

"Hey, freshman. How tall are you?"

Lie. "Six-two."

"Stop it."

Busted. "Okay, six one and a little bit."

"Whatever. You want to try out?"

"Yup."

"Did you row in high school?"

"Nope."

"What did you do?"

"Hoops."

"That's it?"

"Yup. I work hard though."

"Okay, whatever you say. Tomorrow at four."

"At the boathouse?"

"No, freshman. At the track."

"Why the track?"

They didn't answer. The next day, forty kids showed up. The workout was called "The Chief." Five minutes straight of air squats, pushups, burpees, crunches, and high knees running in place. Five sets, with a minute in between. A compact, but brutal, half-hour. The next day, less than half as many kids showed up.

Day two consisted of fifty laps up and down the stadium stairs at the football field—a grueling hour, unlike any workout I'd ever done before. Half the kids didn't finish. The ones that did found themselves hardly able to walk the next morning. Once again, the group shrunk. That's when I realized the coaches didn't need to *pick* anyone. They relied on simple attrition. Brilliant. On the third day, the remaining ten of us joined the actual recruits, another batch of guys who'd rowed through high school. Each was taller, fitter, and laughing at the walk-ons limping after just two workouts.

I spent a lot of my time on schoolwork and most of my energy with the new sport. But it was hard not to notice all the fraternity parties going on in my first semester. From what I could tell, there weren't any other social activities going. Inebriation was assimilation, it seemed. After a couple weeks of going to bed early and hearing the fun pass me by, I went to a party with a couple kids from my floor. I didn't plan on having anything to drink, I just didn't want to miss out on making new friends.

Freshmen were allowed in, but we had to pay a toll—a "quick six" at the bottom of the basement stairs. Six beers, downed as fast as you could. The Sigma brother guarding the basement was huge, almost as wide as the whole stairway. No one could slink around him unnoticed.

He stared, waiting for me to either knock back the six beers or turn my body sideways and shamefully skulk my way back upstairs.

"Are you in or out, freshman?" the giant hollered. "These beers aren't drinking themselves!"

I said I wasn't gonna do this. I already learned the hard way. But there's twenty motherfuckers behind me right now watching. Fuck it. Just get it over with.

So I swiftly paid the price of admission to my first frat party. I got some high-fives from a few older guys that saw how quickly I'd hurled the beers down my gullet. Once those first six were in me, I craved more and more throughout the night, which roared by in a blur.

That was the first time I drank in college—and it would be a Rubicon.

Chapter 2 - Sing the Body Electric

Over the first year, in the backdrop of three-hour crew practices and the buzz of making new friends at parties, something changed inside me. Every few days, waves of guilt and sadness started to ebb and flow through me, like big, weighty pendulum swings. I didn't know what triggered them. I suspected, though, that they weren't a common, shared experience. I felt that I was on this island alone.

Throughout my adolescence, other kids always seemed to be just a bit happier than me. I'd always known and accepted that I was a little different that way. But these swings were a new phenomenon entirely—less of a mood and more like a voice in my head. When it hit me, the laughter and jabber in the room suddenly faded out. In its place, the voice emerged. *You're stupid, useless, and weak. A fucking fake.*

When the pendulum swung, I felt frozen. Shrouded in something heavy and thick. Talking to people was overwhelming. Getting myself up for practice or class felt dreadful. I became burdened by the weightiness of showering or doing my laundry. Most of all, though, was the nasty, raw self-loathing. I felt suddenly as if the space I occupied in the universe was stolen and undeserved.

A reality was becoming clear—I felt bad much more often than I felt good. And when I felt bad, it wasn't simply a mood. The spells seemed elemental, as if they lacked a beginning, middle, or end. And they were crippling—I couldn't focus on homework or talk with friends. I used the alcohol that I'd just gotten reacquainted with to make myself feel better. And at Dartmouth it was wherever I needed it to be—the perfect medicine for a growing, yet unrecognized depression.

Sober, I felt like an ill-fitting puzzle piece. But drunk, I felt a visceral bond with everything and everyone around me. When I was eight drinks in, a deep breath of cold, winter air felt euphoric. After twelve, an embrace with a new friend sent an awesome torrent of companionship through my body. Sixteen, and I felt certain I'd never been happier.

So, with each semester, I ceded more and more ground to this growing habit. The new beginning that I had planned for myself—the one with Walt Whitman readings on the quad—didn't coalesce. It was beer and shots that sang my body electric instead. I ended up joining a fraternity, even after swearing I wouldn't. It was an easy sell for a budding, young drunk.

And I always binged. I drank as much as I could, every time. If alcohol ran out, I didn't stop. I just relocated myself and found more. I never wanted a few beers. I wanted dozens. I came to define the act of drinking as getting drunk to the point of unconsciousness and nothing less. Alcohol wasn't just an accessory to me. It was the thing missing from my body.

So much had changed inside me since I'd arrived. I'd known that person I wanted to be when I stepped off the bus. I saw him—the quintessential student or whatever he was—up close and life-sized. I almost stepped into his silhouette and became him. But I never could. Instead, a duality grew. On one end of the pendulum swing, I had curiosity and exuberance. But on the other, I had a relentless and crippling sadness. And that schism inside me—it was only just beginning to tear me apart.

Chapter 3 - Ham & Eggs

Some days, I came to class excited and focused. And to rowing practice, cheerful and supercharged. Sometimes even leading the way with contagious enthusiasm and a battery pack full of uncanny, manic energy. Other days, though, I felt isolated, shrouded in angst. I didn't make it to class. And I dragged myself to practice with a smile wrenched onto my face. But whenever we launched our boat into the morning mist, still simmering over the river, I felt good. Suspended above the pervasive isolation.

During a hard practice—which was most of them—I exploded into every workout, drawing out pain in every fiber of my muscles. The burning in my legs and arms and lungs felt good and clean. Sometimes

I'd go hard enough to puke over the side of the gunnels of the boat. That felt good, too, like pulling out a splinter buried in my heel. I found a brief sanctuary underneath all that pain and the shared purpose with my team. It was the only thing, besides alcohol, that gave me a sense of comfort in my own skin. In college, I was my very happiest when I was with the team, sober, and busting my ass.

At the start of each season, our coach told us a story before our first race. "A kid sat down for breakfast with his dad before school one day," he'd open in his slow Southern drawl. "He stared down at his plate, not eating much, still thinking about something his teacher had said the previous day. Finally, he looks up from his plate and says, 'Pop, can I ask you a question?'

"'Yes, son. What is it?' the boy's father said, putting down his newspaper.

"'Yesterday, at school, the teacher was trying to explain the difference between *commitment* and *contribution*. She went on for a while about it, but I still don't understand.'

"Dad leans forward and points at the boy's plate and says, 'Son, take a look back down at your breakfast there. What do you see?'

"'Ham and eggs,' the boy replied.

"'Well, you see, Son, a chicken made a *contribution* to your breakfast. But that pig—now, that pig made a *commitment*.'"

"Row Like Pigs" was our mantra. Our school had famously shitty recruiting, which was the only reason I made the team as a walk-on. Top-ranked high-school rowers were usually six-foot-five and two hundred twenty-five pounds—sinewy, veiny fuckers with legs up to their damn chest. But we were mostly an unimpressive group; Will, my best friend on the team, a buck-seventy-five. Me, six-foot-two *if* I had my Jordans on. The rest—similarly undersized, underweight, or under-experienced. But we busted our asses and we were *fast*.

After a strong enough regular season my senior year, we made the twenty-four-team cut for the National Championships in Camden, New Jersey. Despite losing a couple races early in the season, we stayed focused, committed, and peaked at the right time. By the time we got to Nationals, we were rowing as fast as any of us ever had.

We cruised through the first two rounds easily and advanced to the semi-finals: two six-boat races. The top three from each semi-final would go to the grand final. None of us had ever made the grand final at the national championship. In fact, a Dartmouth team hadn't made it in over a decade.

We drew Cornell, Brown, Harvard, UC Berkeley, and Northeastern in our semi. Harvard was a lock to advance. Same with Berkeley. Both boats were chock full of the veiny, six-foot, five-inch, future olympians. Brown, we knew we could beat, after finishing ahead of them a couple weeks prior. Cornell was just there to give the rest of us their lunch money. That left us and Northeastern. One of us was going on to the big dance. The other, to the showers.

The Northeastern Huskies beat us the first time we met them earlier that season. But a few weeks later, we smoked them in our next matchup. Both crews had something to prove—it was a winner-take-all rubber match. We were locked in, eyes dead ahead, waiting for the starting gun.

Bang.

The silence shattered like glass. Coxswains shouted indecipherable and obscene commands over their loudspeakers. Blades frenetically carved up the water. A few dozen guys tried to pull hard enough to snap their fucking oars in half. By the five-hundred-meter mark, a quarter of the way through the race, Harvard and Cal had started to pull away. Cornell, Brown, Northeastern, and us all sat even. Apparently, Cornell had gotten their shit together.

"We're in the middle thousand meters now! Time to put these fuckers in the rearview!" Kate barked.

The unique pain of rowing leaves no part of the body unscathed. The lactic acid builds up fast—and holy shit does it burn. It starts in the legs, shoots up to the back and arms. That's when the lungs catch fire—a searing pain that only relents when you stop. Even the hands get bloodied, as skin peels away on the wooden handles. But with five hundred meters to go, at least we had something to show for it—Brown and Cornell were indeed in the rearview. *See ya.*

"We just passed the five-hundred-meter mark and we're dead fucking even with Northeastern! On my count, we're taking it up to forty strokes per minute. Ready… now!"

The final five hundred meters lay ahead—about a minute and a half to find out which of us wanted it most. Sixty strokes—each one an invitation to be immortal or to surrender.

"Put these motherfuckers away!" Kate shouted, so loud that the speakers crackled. "Twenty strokes left! I want to… "

The noise faded. *You're always gonna remember this moment if you don't choose courage, right fucking now.* I thought of my team and nothing else. And I gave them everything. After a mile and a quarter of racing neck-and-neck, we beat them out by six feet. Everyone in the boat shouted, shook the shoulders of the guy in front of them, and then collapsed onto the guy behind. I stayed upright for a beat longer, looking down at Pat, who was laying on my shins and wincing in pain. Then, before collapsing onto the bow, I glanced down at the idle water. I was always amused by its indifference to all of us.

When I showed up freshman fall, asking about a tryout, I just thought I might have fun trying something new. I never thought I'd be a captain of the sixth best team in the whole country. I felt the happiest I'd been in years... but it wouldn't last.

I woke up the next morning at six-thirty a.m., distraught. The feeling of accomplishment had already been replaced by that scornful, insidious voice in my head. *You should have trained harder. You shouldn't have drank so much for the past four years. You should have been... better.* In a matter of hours, the satisfaction of achievement diminished under the suffocating distress of shame.

Shame. That was the way. The language I spoke to myself.

Chapter 4 - Lehman, Bro

During my senior year, I mentored teens with chronic illnesses every few days after class through a local program I found. Gary had a tumor in his brain when he was a child. To remove it, they cut through his hypothalamus, which regulates appetite. He recovered from the surgery, but it left him permanently feeling like he hadn't eaten for days. By sixteen, he'd grown to over four hundred pounds.

His parents and the program hoped that I could get him to work out. But he was petrified, both by the anticipation of immense physical discomfort as well as the self-consciousness about how he looked while exercising. He relented, but the stipulation was that we would train at Dartmouth, not his high school, where someone familiar might see him. We started with very, very light jogging on the indoor track. He ran on the inside lane, close to the railing, in case he needed to grab it. He looked miserable, and I felt like a cruel prison guard.

"One, two, three, four! Almost there, just a little bit more! Five, six, seven, eight! Man, oh man, you're doing great!" I hollered, making shit up just to try and get him to smile.

After a few weeks he wasn't as terrified before each workout. And he wasn't quitting in the middle or even stopping for a break. During a jog one day, Gary suddenly let out a primal, guttural yell and picked up his pace. I was so fired up that I just screamed right back at him. It was his fastest mile yet, by far.

"That was fucking awesome, Gary! Great work!" I shouted at the finish, squeezing him with a big hug.

"Thanks. I don't know what came over me. I just got—excited. I feel happy right now. For the first time in forever."

"Fuck yeah, dude. I'm so proud of you."

It wasn't always that easy. Sometimes he skipped our meetings, turned off his phone, and disappeared. I got worried the first time. I thought maybe I pushed him too hard. But his mom told me that it happened a lot, and to try C&A's Pizza on Main Street. Sure enough, that's where I found both him and the remnants of an extra-large sausage and pepperoni. He got mad at himself afterwards and said he wanted to quit. I told him to forgive himself and that it wasn't a step backwards if he took two steps forward.

Gary eventually got into college. He was terrified of moving away from home and scared of what new peers would think and say about his body. But just like in the gym, he courageously decided to go for it. After we celebrated, I reminded him that high school kids were *way* worse.

I didn't work with Gary and the others—like Jamie who had Crohn's disease and Carla with diabetes—just to pay some penance. That was part of it, to be sure. But it went deeper. Helping Gary battle his own demons motivated me. I related to it. I understood wanting to shrink, hide, and give up. But if I could help him chip away at the shame he felt, maybe it would remind me to do the same. So, when I graduated, I knew I wanted to keep working with kids. It made me feel good. It quieted that mean, excoriating voice in my head.

I felt self-conscious stepping into the auditorium and seeing all the little career fair booths set up. I wore whatever rags I normally meandered around campus in. Meanwhile, other kids sported blazers and chinos, hunting down recruiters from Mackenzie, Goldman Sachs, and Lehman Brothers, still very much in its heyday.

I finally made my way to a far corner of the auditorium, where all the lonely, underpopulated nonprofits sat clustered together. One table caught my eye. A modest banner read *Eckerd Youth Alternatives*. The brochures had pictures of teenagers and counselors in a campsite.

"Are you thinking about social work?" the rep asked, giving me the warmest of smiles.

"Wait—I thought this was Lehman Brothers? Just kidding. Yes, I am. What's Eckerd?"

"We're a wilderness-based residential treatment facility for at-risk and incarcerated teenage boys. We have camps all over the East Coast. There's one not too far, in Rhode Island."

"Residential? So, do you guys, like, live there with the kids you work with?"

"Yup, that's right."

"And the kids... how at-risk *are* they? Like, sneaking into the movies or..."

She laughed. Then, seeming to know the words that would resonate inside of me, she said, "I wish. My first two years at Eckerd were the hardest thing I've ever done. The kids challenged me more than I ever thought possible. And—" She let a pause hang for a moment. "I'd do it all over again."

Out of nowhere, my eyes welled up. I didn't anticipate it nor fully understand why. I shook her hand and took a pamphlet from her—the only one I took that day. It stayed with me as I packed my dorm up after graduation, shoveled four years of crap in the back of my 1987 Suburban, and drove back to the Bay Area with Alex and James, two of my best friends. When I returned home, I slept on it one more night, alone and sober. I woke up with a clear sense of purpose.

"I'm in," I said to the recruiter.

"That's terrific. You won't regret it, and you'll make such an impact, I can already tell."

She slotted me in the fall training session at their Rhode Island facility. In the meantime, I took a couple of months off, with no school or work.

It should have been a fun summer break.

Chapter 5 - Eight Bit

The spells started getting worse. They became sharper in intensity, and they lasted much longer. I couldn't make a meal, take a shower, or even leave the house. I couldn't hold conversations. The voice of someone standing right in front of me would fade into the background, drowned out by the voice inside. *You're weird. Scared. Fucking pathetic.* For days, even up to a week, I stayed trapped in my room and in my head.

But then, like dull clouds clearing the sky to reveal the bright, crisp sun, I'd feel euphoric, touched by the magnificence of everything. A favorite Guns N' Roses song would electrify me. I'd be whisked to the front row, center stage, hearing Axl wail "November Rain." A run through the park was a visceral exultation. I'd finish, stretch my arms up towards the sky and be mesmerized by the power of the human body.

I couldn't sleep during these euphoric episodes. But I didn't want to. Sleep was just hours of life wasted, I thought. I wanted to do everything. Be everywhere. Talk to everyone. I called my friends every day and night, chattering in hyper-speed. They had to tell me to slow down because they couldn't follow whatever I was yapping on about. I ran up my credit cards without regard, buying clothes that I didn't need. I drank, smoked, did drugs, and slept with any girl that gave me the time of day. But just like depression, euphoria passed too, leaving me tired, empty, and on the brink of more despair.

And so, all summer, the pendulum swung back and forth. I knew something was wrong, but I didn't do anything or tell anyone. When I was euphoric, I was too swept up by the sensations to care. And when I was depressed, I was too paralyzed to act. All I could do was drink to numb the pain and wait for it to pass. I figured I could endure whatever was happening to me until it went away.

I woke up one morning at Alex's apartment in San Francisco. I'd gotten in the habit of doing a systems-check on my mind once my eyes opened to see if I felt up, down, or, hopefully, even-keel. As if my head was an old 8-bit Nintendo, I didn't know what I was going to get when it turned on. I left the city with my mind feeling as normal as I could hope for. On top of that, there was no traffic and it wasn't even foggy in San Fran. Yeah… all too good to be true.

In an instant, when I was halfway over the Bay Bridge, the calm, idyllic morning was obliterated. Without a warning or a trigger, my mind exploded into a thousand shards of glass. I lost all order, reason, and sequence. Nonsensical thoughts raced in sharp, crisscrossing directions. Indecipherable, shrieking noise. *Everyone thinks I am awful. My shoes are all scuffed. Ruined. I'm going nowhere. In life. Speed up to a hundred. Blood, bone, guts.* I couldn't reason with myself or calm myself down. Within minutes, I was certain that I had gone insane. And then, with just as much certainty—*being dead would be better than this.*

I wanted to steer myself into the guard rail and fly over the edge into the bay. My reeling mind and a basic survival instinct battled back and forth for control of the steering wheel until I got myself home. I sobbed uncontrollably for the rest of the day, until I was exhausted enough to fall asleep. I woke up in the deepest, heaviest depression yet.

I didn't go outside the house for three or four days. Leaving my bed, taking showers, and brushing my teeth were arduous, uphill climbs. Food was nauseating. Talking to a person was as nerve-wracking as speaking to a packed auditorium, so I avoided everyone and didn't answer my phone. Exercising, reading, going to the store—all were off the table.

Thoughts of death and dying ripped through my mind all day. I imagined flinging my car off that bridge and smacking the water with no seatbelt—my face shredding through the splintered windshield. Or nestling a gun in the divot of my chest and a sending bullet screaming into me—my hands red from the blood racing through my fingers. Dark and gruesome images ran on an endless slideshow. I had no power. No ability to stop them.

I was supposed to leave in a few days for Rhode Island. I couldn't imagine how I would even get to the airport, much less begin an intense two-week training. The night before I left, I prayed—to a God I didn't know and who didn't know me—that I might snap out of the depression before the sun rose. But He or She or They were not listening.

I couldn't see a way through all the usually mundane obstacles in front me. The subway to the airport, the security lines, the ticketing agents. The small spaces I would have to fit into. The crowds of people everywhere. Rushing and pushing and shouting and grabbing. It all seemed unbearable. I wished I could rewind a few hours to when I was still asleep and hit pause there, forever. The only thing propelling me forward was the guilt I'd feel if I quit. Letting down some people I hadn't even met yet.

One thing at a time. Just pack a bag. I threw handfuls of clothes into a duffel bag until it was full. I couldn't think clearly enough to make sure it was the right stuff. I'd have to buy whatever I forgot when I got there.

Next, call a cab. I hoped that the driver didn't speak one word to me on the drive the entire trip to SFO. *They always want to talk, talk, talk.* Fortunately, not that day.

Go to the counter. Check in. Be normal. The departures area was a terrifying, chaotic maze. People zoomed by me in a blur, yapping frantically into their phones, hurriedly shoving last-minute shit into their bags and crappy food into their faces.

Security. Fuck. I knew the questions that the agents would ask. I knew the documents they would need to see. I even knew how to take my shoes and belt off and slide a couple plastic tubs through the X-ray machine. But I thought I would fuck something up and get pulled out of line and sent into a dark room. *What if there's a gun in my bag? Maybe someone put one in my bag to get me arrested?*

But, at last, I made it to my airplane seat. Quiet and stillness for a few hours. I waited until the drink cart, crawling an inch at a time through the aisles, finally got to me. *Ten fucking dollars for a tiny bottle of Jack?* But it could have been a hundred bucks—I'd have paid. I needed to breathe and to sleep.

I landed in Providence late at night. The city was quiet with empty streets. I felt a visceral relief to get away from the commotion of the airport and the tight confines of the plane. I found a bar near my hotel and drank some more. I tried to distract myself with ESPN highlights on their TV, but I just stared through the screen.

The next morning, training began. I couldn't hear what my instructors or the other trainees were saying. Couldn't focus on their words. I only heard my own voice in my head, telling me I wasn't prepared for this job. That I was too messed up to help these kids. That I might be losing my fucking mind. That I needed a drink. *Make sure they can't tell. Fake it for as long as you have to.*

For a couple weeks, I wore the mask of someone normal. I laughed when the group laughed. I followed the group when it moved. I mimicked during role plays and drills. Nighttime was easier. After the full days, I was tired enough for the frantic pace of my thoughts to finally slow. And, with everyone asleep, the strain of interactions was put on hold. I stayed up late, alone, because I cherished those precious minutes. I knew that, once I fell asleep, my mind wouldn't belong to me again until the next night.

The episode was long and grueling. I wanted to run away and escape. But I kept myself tethered to the ground by thinking about the job. *This is where you wanted to be. Here. Helping these kids. So don't fucking quit on them.* After a couple of weeks, just before training finished, the depression finally released its nasty grip on me. I convinced myself that I'd beaten it, as if it was like chicken pox and ran its course once, never to be heard from again.

Right—as if it was fucking chicken pox.

Part Three

Chapter 1 - Kumbaya

I'd been oblivious to the beauty of my new surroundings. Deep in the woods of Rhode Island, we were buried in red and yellow foliage and surrounded by streams, rocks, and trails. It resembled, at least for a while, the brochure I picked up at the career fair.

We had three campsites, each made up of mulch-laden paths and small cabins that the kids and counselors built themselves. Every campsite housed one group of about ten boys, along with two counselors, called chiefs. Between the three campsites sat dining halls, recreation fields, and a big, murky pond. We called it a "lake" because we swam in it and swimming in a "pond" didn't sound right.

The camp directors asked us to make a two-year minimum commitment. But I only knew my first co-counselor for three weeks. He split after one of the boys tried to hotwire his car. The next one left after she got punched in the face. On and on, the carousel went. Most of the chiefs had a social work background or a wealth of volunteer experience. But *none* of us had ever done anything like this.

The boys were all at-risk, or they'd already been incarcerated and were finishing their sentence at our camp. Some came from households rampant with drug and alcohol addiction. Others, with physical or sexual abuse. Some were taken from homes left empty after their parents had been locked up. Whatever their background, our goal was to teach them the behaviors needed for lasting reentry into homes, schools, and communities.

We used a wilderness-based therapy model. A high-risk proposition, to be sure. When it worked, they'd make their own dinner, chop wood, and even build cabins. But sometimes, those axes turned into projectiles instead of tools. Sometimes the kids ran away, jumped each other, or assaulted counselors. And sometimes, when all hell had broken loose, kids were dragged into the back of police cars and returned to jail.

One night, a fight broke out between groups in the dining hall. Someone in one group whispered something to a boy in another when he walked by. They had outside beef prior to camp—rival neighborhood gangs. First came the whisper. Then a shove. Then a thrown plate from a third boy. In less than a minute, twenty boys were kicking, punching, and hurling whatever they could get their hands on.

We managed to corral them out of the dining hall and away from sharp utensils, metal corners, and the kitchen staff. The staff were trained to make fantastic chicken-parm, but not to put kids into submission holds. The fight continued outside, where they had rocks to throw, sticks to swing, and the dark of night to hide in.

While I stood between a few small groups, arms outstretched, trying to keep them separated, a boy named Marcus eyed us from about fifty feet out and up a slight hill. Usually, Marcus stayed out of trouble unless someone provoked him. Then, he became a mad pit-bull off his leash. From his perch, he bent over and picked up a grapefruit-sized rock resting at his feet. Most kids would have picked a smaller rock. But Marcus was as strong as anyone there—including the counselors—and could launch it with ease.

In the dark, the rock disappeared as soon as it left his hand. No one but me saw him launch it. I stood frozen, unable to get myself or any of the boys out of the way of something I couldn't see. I could only hope. After a few long seconds, I heard the small boulder whiz by my ear, inches away from cratering my skull. Amidst the noise and the dark, no one else even knew what had just happened. The group I was wrangling up just kept barking back and forth at each other, unaware that Marcus could have just landed me—or one of them— in the ICU.

The next day, I pulled him aside. I told him he could have killed someone, that he needed to stop and think, even if he was angry. He told me that whenever he got that mad, it felt like a blackout. No memory of what he'd done. He said it started after the years of countless beatings he and his mom endured. He finally snapped one night and bashed his step dad's face in with a can of chili. That's how he landed in jail in the first place.

The trauma many of the boys endured had created angry, violent, and unpredictable teens. Some of them acted out every day, releasing their pain one small outburst at a time. Others had pain resting deeper beneath the surface. Their episodes were less frequent, but more intense. And then came Juan, whose pain was something entirely different.

Chapter 2 - Juan

Juan landed in my group after bouncing in and out of juvenile hall for years. He had an infectious smile and magnetic personality. The other boys were all drawn to him, immediately ushering him to the top of their pecking order. He was the smallest in our group, but by far the strongest and fastest. He ran a deadly deep route on the football field, pulled a nasty crossover on the court, and was flat-out uncatchable in capture-the-flag.

My group had been struggling. I had some tough kids who didn't give a shit whether they got out or not. Juan said he wanted to use our program to finally get himself out of the system. And I believed, at the time, that he did. We quickly reached an agreement: I would help him get released as early as possible, and he'd use his popularity—and daunting reputation—to help me get the group's behaviors in check. And, of course, we'd also join up together during capture-the-flag, laying waste to the other team.

The other kids did whatever Juan said, even the worst actors. All he had to do was tell them to quit fucking around, and they suddenly became little angels. After a week or two, he achieved what I'd been trying to do for months. I thought they followed him because they revered him. And they did, to an extent. The personality, the big grin, the athleticism—it was all magnetic stuff. But I realized soon enough that they feared him, too.

After his first few weeks—a honeymoon period—I saw flashes of a ferocious temper. He could only keep himself in check for so long when someone got on his nerves. When other kids kept the group from getting to a meal on time or held up his bedtime, he'd sometimes punish instead of lead. Giving a quick shot to the ribs was easier—and quicker—than building consensus. I started to think I'd been had. Maybe his good behavior was just an act.

Juan's release date came up after about six months. By then, after more and more violent, manipulative tendencies, I felt ready for him to leave. But I wondered if he actually wanted to go home. Over our time together, I'd learned about his dad, the monster waiting for him after his release from our custody. Juan had told me that if he talked back, he'd have to kneel on uncooked rice while holding a phonebook over his head. If he came home late, he would catch the belt. And, sometimes, he and his sister just got roughed up for no reason at all.

He'd worked hard to get himself out, or at least played the part. But on the brink of it, he may have decided that he'd just be trading one prison for another. Perhaps he'd be better off locked up, where at least he wouldn't be a victim of someone else's violence. Instead, he could be the afflicter.

A week before his release date, in the middle of the night, he went on a rampage. He ran through the campsite, peppering anyone he came across with punches and kicks—even some who thought they were his friends. No one fought back—they were terrified by the crazed desperation in his eyes. We tried to catch him, but he dipped in-between us like an elusive running back.

I'd loaned him my favorite sweatshirt a few days earlier when he was cold. It was a black hoodie, five sizes too big for him, with *Cal State Long Beach* embroidered in yellow on the chest. The next time he darted near me, I leaped and stretched out like a rangy defensive end. My fingers clutched the back of my own sweatshirt, and I took him down. The police were already on the way. He scratched and clawed until he heard the sirens pull up. Then his body went still. He gave me a menacing smile, with the red and blue strobe lights bouncing off his teeth and eyes.

"This is what you wanted, isn't it?" I asked. He responded with only that unsettling grin.

I held him down until the cops took over. They handcuffed him, pressed his head down, and chucked him in the back of their squad car. He left in my sweatshirt. I hoped he'd keep it and remember that someone had cared and tried to help him.

Many years later, I found out he'd been arrested on murder charges. The news said he stabbed his sister's ex-boyfriend to death. Not long after, he was killed in prison.

Chapter 3 - Five Foot Nothin'

Only two chiefs remained from our training class: me and Chief Annie. In fact, Annie had been abandoned by even more coworkers than me. One afternoon, a kid in her group, Eric, pestered another, Mario, by throwing little sticks and pebbles at his feet. Mario, easily the biggest kid at camp, gave the smaller Eric a very generous warning period. Eric was about Annie's size, barely five feet tall and a hundred pounds, and was gunning for an ass-kicking. After the third or fourth rock landed on his foot, Mario's eyes narrowed, his fists tensed, and he took flight.

I ran towards Mario to intercept him. But before I could even get there, Annie flung herself at him and wrapped her arms around one of his legs. She barely slowed him down. He dragged her along with him until, after seeing his counselor clasped to his calf, his temper ebbed. Eric escaped, unscathed, while Mario and I helped Chief Annie up to her feet.

I hadn't talked much with Annie before that incident, only helping her group for a few days because her co-counselor had just quit. But by the time I went back over to my own group, I was awestruck. *That girl is fucking badass*, I thought. And that was Annie—resilient and dedicated, even if it put her in harm's way.

Our shifts were twenty-four hours, five days a week. On our two days off, chiefs retreated to the house we all shared. Maybe because our bosses knew we were about the same age, or maybe because they saw me look at her a certain kind of way, my time off mysteriously changed to the same days as Annie's.

On our first night off together, we got hammered at the nearby tavern. We ate greasy bar food, drank draught beer, and crammed in as much life story as we could. She was from Canada, adored Dave Matthews Band, and had wanted a Jeep Wrangler since she was a kid—which she'd finally gotten with some graduation money. I came from Oakland, adored the Golden State Warriors, and drove a 1987 Chevy Suburban, which I'd recently careened into a tree after the first snow.

"Look, in Cali, nobody taught us how to drive in the damn snow, okay?" I pleaded.

"Well, you start by putting it in four-wheel drive."

"Is that what that extra lever thing is for?"

"Oh, brother."

"Let's go skiing tomorrow. I'll use the four-wheel drive this time."

We'd have to leave in about three hours, tired and hungover like hell. I was ambivalent, but I'd do it. Mainly, I just wanted to see whether she'd turn down a dare.

"Fuck yes," she said.

Shit. "All right, you're on," I said, giving her a glare. "And you'd better not bail."

"Oh, don't worry about me," she teased. "I'm leaving at five a.m., with or without you."

"Sheesh. Okay, okay, five-thirty it is."

We were at Dunkin' by the time dawn broke. We ordered two extra-large Extra-Extras. Enough caffeine to fire up a lawn mower, and enough cream and sugar to make a milkshake.

With some coffee in me, I asked her, "So, I'm curious—how exactly did you end up here at the camp? I know you wanted to work with foster kids. But, like, there are easier places to do it."

"This is a pretty bad answer, but it just sort of happened," she said.

"Ha! Yeah, not a great answer."

"I came across this place last year before graduation and—I don't know—I just couldn't really put it out of my mind. And I just felt like I was supposed to do it. So here I am."

"Wow."

"Yeah, I told you it was a bad answer."

"No, I mean, that's basically why I'm here."

"Well, I'm happy we both showed up, because I don't know who else I'd hang out with."

We got to the Vermont ski resort before the gaggles of ski-schooling children and stoned, teenage snowboarders rolled in. The sun had just crested over the mountain by the time we snapped into our skis for the first run. The weather felt crisp, but comfortable—perfect for this unusual first date.

I usually liked hitting black diamonds, moguls, and working up a sweat. But that day was relaxed and idyllic. We spent as much time sipping coffee and smoking cigarettes at the lounge as we spent on the slopes themselves. When we actually tried getting our money's worth for the lift tickets, the old resort's creaky chair lifts were so slow that we just kept talking and talking.

"So, do you think you'll stay at camp for the whole two-years?" she asked.

"Well, in general, I usually try not to quit stuff. Including these delightful cigarettes."

"Okay, but seriously, I imagine all the counselors who've left have said the same thing. I've had two quit already. And you're on your third. What if that just ends up being us?"

"Well, I'm not gonna lie," I admitted, "I don't think I could have imagined dealing with some of this shit. It's intense. And I didn't think there would be so many axes! Why the axes? Can't we just use Duraflames?"

"Right!? Let's teach them the different kinds of knots instead of chopping wood."

With the top of the lift in sight, I put my toe in the water. "Well, I think it'll be easier with you here. I really like hanging out together."

"I'm feeling the same way." Then she turned and looked at me, right before she hopped off the lift. "I'll stick it out if you do."

I almost forgot to slide off the chair.

The sun felt warmer on my cheeks for the rest of the day. The fizzy excitement of finding a high school crush charged through me, along with a certain hope for the future that I hadn't felt in a long time.

On the way home, I fucked up the directions. Big time. But neither of us noticed we were halfway to Albany, NY, until we saw a huge sign that said, *Welcome to the Empire State.* We spent ten hours in the car that night. But we didn't mind at all. We just dove into conversation, which quickly evolved from bantering to confiding.

I told her about my dad. How I used to run scared through our own house. The time after my fifteenth birthday when he pulled out a butcher's knife, pointed it at his chest, and demanded to know why I wanted to hurt them. She told me about losing her virginity. Without consent. Blacked out, to a stranger at a bar while she was on a vacation. Pushing him away and saying, "No," to no avail.

"I'm so sorry."

"It's okay. I think I'm stronger because of it," she said, with a conviction that gave me chills.

I felt a raw, primal anger. I'd barely known Annie for a couple months. Yet, when she told me about the rape, I suddenly saw my hands tightening around this unknown animal's throat until he never got even a sip of air again. It might have been only one night and a ski trip, so far, but I knew this feeling was something different. The beginning of a crazy, wild kind of love. The kind that would make me want to destroy anything that ever hurt her.

When we finally got home—by way of upstate New York—we climbed the stairs to her room. It was like we already knew each other's bodies and the rhythm of each other's heartbeats. Once we'd stripped down to nothing and ripped the covers off her bed, we paused for a moment. We each took a few deep breaths, momentarily resisting the gravity pulling us towards one another. I looked into her eyes. She, mine. And we stayed still for several seconds. The connection was absolute and irresistible. And then, when the gravity finally overwhelmed us, we surrendered to it fully.

From that night on, we spent as much time together as possible. Our time off together was perfect. Dreamlike. When the weather was nice, we visited everywhere the state of Rhode Island had to offer, albeit a pretty short list. When it rained or snowed, we stayed in bed all day and tried not to check the time. At work, we slipped by each other's cabins late at night to drop off handwritten letters, because our cell phones didn't work in the woods. And, 'cause it was cute.

While other counselors quit left and right, Annie and I gave each other the strength to keep going. After the worst weeks, which we spent deflecting everything from swear words to projectiles, two days together renewed our waning motivation. Annie's fierce reluctance to quit rivaled my own tenacity. She had the strength to try to wrestle a two-hundred-pound juvenile to the ground before he beat the piss out of a smaller kid. The strength to hold together a splintered family. And the strength to persevere, and love again, after the most vile transgression. Annie was the soul mate I didn't know was out there for me. I was falling, fast. It didn't take me long to know I wanted to be around her forever.

Chapter 4 - Brandon

Brandon was sixteen when he arrived at the camp. In the middle of robbing a house, he discovered the owner was inside. He panicked and cracked the guy with a bat. After a year of jail time for burglary and assault, authorities transferred him over to us. The rate of recidivism—going back to jail—was much higher among the older boys. At that age, many had already joined gangs, dropped out of school, or left their homes. Realistic treatment goals for them at our program were often reduced to physical safety and eating three squares a day. But with Brandon, more felt possible, like he could be one of the kids that defy the statistics. Annie and I made it our mission.

But bad influence waited everywhere. Rhode Island was tiny. These guys had all come from the same few neighborhoods, and many already knew one another. Fights often broke out over some preexisting beef. If they had no beef, they recruited each other to join their gangs. As hard as we tried to steer them toward a diploma or GED, someone else tried to pull them into the street life. Brandon, with his reputation for knocking guys out with bats, was a five-star recruit.

Miguel was almost eighteen and had been in a gang since dropping out of high school. Fully filled out, he stood over six feet tall. He had tattoos on his chest, arms, and neck, scrawling out his gang letters in Olde English characters. Like Juan, Miguel intimidated the other boys. When he pulled one under his wing, we had a hard time breaking his spell. We couldn't wait for him to turn eighteen and just get the fuck out of there. In the meantime, we had to keep him away from Brandon.

Kids in different groups weren't allowed to talk, so they resorted to sneaking notes to each other in the communal dining hall instead. They'd get up from their group's table and head to the bathroom, where they could briefly get out of sight, and leave rolled up pieces of paper under the soap dispenser or inside a roll of toilet paper. It wasn't exactly tradecraft. But we usually let them think they had outsmarted us, just to keep them from finding better hiding places.

We checked the bathroom between turns and easily found their stealthy missives. Most contained asinine enough messages, so we just put them back where we found them. We only intercepted it if they were planning something—a fight, a runaway, or even a late-night heist in the kitchen. But, far more often, someone was just lying about hooking up with a girl back home.

The last two kids we wanted passing notes back and forth were Miguel and Brandon. One, our consummate bad apple. The other, our best chance at a real success story. When we saw Brandon use the bathroom right after Miguel, we didn't think it was a coincidence.

After dinner, Annie and I pulled him out of the group. She demanded an answer while I stood with my arms crossed. "Brandon, what was that?"

"What was *what*?"

"Come on, dude. Don't be cute," I said. "What did that note say?"

His face got a bit red.

"Oh, you thought we didn't see? You're Jason Bourne, now? Seriously, tell us what's going on."

"What do you think? Miguel wants to jump me into his gang when I get out."

"Why would you want to do that?" Annie asked.

"He lives a few blocks from me. If I say no, the same dudes that would have had my back are gonna be trying to beat *my* ass. So, what's the difference. Fucked up, either way."

"Let the dude find some other motherfucker, man!" I said, before grabbing him hard by both shoulders and pulling him closer. "When you get back out there, you can be somebody, man. You can do something. Some of these kids don't have a fuckin' chance. But you do, for real."

He looked back at me, motionless, like my grip was propping him up.

"But not if you don't finish high school. Not if you join a gang with fucking Miguel. Not if you end up back in jail—or worse."

Brandon's expression got serious. "What the fuck do you know? You're not from where I'm from."

I realized I'd pushed too hard. "You're right, I'm not. And I'm sorry if I crossed a line. It's just that… we just know what you're capable of and who you could become."

The defensiveness relaxed a bit. "Just let me just think about all this shit. Damn, I honestly don't know why you care so much. But I appreciate you."

We didn't have a lot of kids like Brandon. Sometimes, we found it hard to stay motivated, knowing that most of the kids would end up back on the street until they found their way to jail again. But if we could help even one of the boys turn his life around, it would all be worth it. And we hoped Brandon might be the one. So, we maintained a steady pressure on him every day after that. We reminded him to do his homework, be a leader, and, for fuck's sake, stay the hell away from Miguel.

Brandon might have been our best hope, but we gave each kid our all. Late one night, after everyone was down, little Eric, the same one Mario almost vaporized, took off toward the highway. When I caught up to him, I found him sitting on a log, smoking a cigarette he'd somehow snuck into camp. He started to run again when he saw me, but I quickly wrapped my arms around him and put him gently on his butt. When he finally stopped squirming, I kept him embraced in a hug for a few seconds.

"Tell me what's wrong," I told him.

"What do you even care? You're just going to take me back to the group."

"Yeah, I am. You're right. But not yet. For now, I'm just here to listen. We can sit here as long as you want," I said, slowly. "But you can't smoke those cigarettes. Sorry, bud."

After he half-heartedly stomped out the smoldering cigarette in some dry sticks and leaves, he said, "Everyone else has somewhere to go. I don't."

It was nearing the holidays. Most of the kids were able to go home for a few days on probation to see their families. But Eric's dad was long gone, and his single mother lost custody years prior. After he got out of camp, he'd just go back to his group home.

"Okay, let's talk about that. But first, why don't you make sure that cigarette is all the way out, so we don't start a forest fire?"

He smiled a bit as he stomped it again with his loose, untied hiking boots, a bit more attentively than the first time around.

"I hear you, Eric, and I'm so sorry," I said. "But you know what, little man?" I said as I put my arm around him. "We care about you here and will try to make Christmas special as best we can."

I didn't rush him back to bed. I waited until he tired himself out from crying. When I felt his little body pass out and lean into mine, I nudged him awake and walked him back to bed at about three in the morning. I went to my cabin and had a bit of whiskey to help myself get to sleep before my alarm went off at six. Annie and I were scheduled to take one of the groups on a canoe trip that morning.

I should have been exhausted when I woke up after late nights like that. But I never was. The surges of energy that regularly zipped through me took the place of rest or nourishment. At seven a.m., I trotted down to the campsite hooting and hollering with a coffee in one hand and a canoe paddle in the other. The boys were groggy and petulant, but Annie and I had them piled into the van by eight.

The trip was a delightful shitshow. Eric tried to stand in his canoe and got whacked by a low hanging tree branch, sending him head-first into the river. Then Kevin and Jamal tried jousting with their paddles. Their asses promptly ended up in the river, too. Not to be outdone, Jonathan swallowed a little frog on a dare. Neither Annie nor I saw that one, or we would have stopped him… maybe.

Out on the river, a youthful innocence seeped out of the boys' otherwise hardened demeanors. There was no gangster, tough guy bullshit. They were just a bunch of kids. Splashing. Laughing. The carefree stuff of summer camp. A rare moment that made the chaos and trauma we lived in with these boys feel immeasurably worthwhile.

Chapter 5 - Coffee Break

As far as my supervisors were concerned, I was doing a bang-up job. I was able and willing to stay awake all night with a kid who tried to run away and then lead a group on a canoe trip the next morning. Nothing looked wrong on the outside, so they didn't question how I did it. They didn't know I hardly slept. That I drank to quiet my thoughts down enough to get any sleep at all. They didn't know that sometimes I had irrational, obsessive fears that I would hurt the kids or abduct them.

They made me the supervisor for all the groups after a year. Sometimes, they had me work ten-day or fifteen-day shifts if they needed coverage. When counselors quit or needed a vacation, they had me plug the holes. During those stretches, sometimes I'd run a group with no co-counselor. It should have been exhausting, not to mention precarious. But I really didn't mind. I liked the nutty challenge of running groups by myself.

A counselor bailed one night without warning. He packed up his stuff and just split. No two-week notice. Shit, not even two-hour notice. His co-counselor had recently left, too, so we literally had no one to run this particularly tough group. My boss called and said they needed me to skip my time off and take over until they had a replacement.

The kids reveled in their successful mutiny and refused to go down the first night. They howled and cackled in the dark while throwing rocks and logs around the campsite. Some even climbed up the cabins, tearing the vinyl windows and siding along the way. They all wanted to see my reaction. Would I ignore them and give up for the night? Pack my bags and run for the hills, like the last chief? Or maybe find someone to come help me?

"What are you going to do, Chief Dave? Get out your radio and call for some backup?" one goaded, while the rest still howled and jeered.

I stared right at him, yanked the radio out of my backpack, and ripped out the battery. The boys all knew the radios were our lifeline to more support—or even the police, if needed. But it was also *their* lifeline if food or supplies were out. I chucked the battery into the woods, slammed the radio into the dirt, and shouted, "It's just you and me for the next ten days! That's it! No one is coming to help me. But guess what? No one is coming to help *you, either*! So, no, I don't need the fucking radio."

It was a reckless move. A game of chicken with a dozen juveniles who had just been howling at the damn moon.

"Yo, Chief Dave is real, dog. This motherfucker ain't playing!" another said, while the rest seconded.

We crushed it for the next week and a half. Our campsite sparkled clean. We arrived on time for meals and activities. The kids even did the math and reading assignments, usually used as kindling for the fireplaces in their tents. They liked performing well, they just hadn't realized it before. They had grown accustomed to others viewing them as menaces and so they just acted the part. To them, praise and encouragement wasn't a familiar language. But when they heard it, they glowed. My bosses were ecstatic. They hated dealing with this usually uncontrollable group and its revolving cast of counselors. And I felt just as happy—I exulted in the challenge of helping these kids find a better version of themselves.

But inside of me, seams unraveled. Though I remained totally immersed in my job, sometimes for twenty hours a day, the voice in my head grew louder. It invaded me, shouting and blurting, impulsively and irrationally. I couldn't make the voice disappear. I could only temporarily drown it out with alcohol. I drank almost every night to quiet my thoughts and fall asleep, only to wake up a few hours later with the same frenetic anxiety as the day before.

Around the kids, I obsessively feared I might do something horrendous. While we chopped wood—*What if I start swinging this ax at them?* If we were out on a day trip—*What if I drive this van off a cliff?* And when I spent time alone with one of them—*What if I am actually a sick, pedophile fuck and try to molest him?*

And when I was alone, my distorted thoughts turned on me. If a car drove by while I walked along the road—*Should I leap in front at the last second? Before it can swerve?* If I saw a knife on another counselor's belt—*How would the blade feel sinking into my chest? Coarse and rough? Or smooth and precise?* If someone stood in front of me talking—*What if their hands were missing? Or a leg?*

Every morning I stopped by the kitchen before seven a.m. to fill my thermos with Pop Dan's black, gritty coffee. Pop Dan, as he was known, was the head cook. He was a tall, chubby guy in his sixties with a bushy, salt-and-pepper beard, which barely concealed a toothy grin stained from coffee and Copenhagen.

"Morning, Dave!" He blurted out, louder than I was ready for. "Cream and sugar?"

"Your coffee is terrible. So yes, of course, cream and fucking sugar."

"Ha! What a pussy!"

Before I could respond to the ever-vulgar, but somehow affable, Pop Dan, I noticed the big butcher's knife behind him on the kitchen counter. In my mind, his arm disappeared. *Blood. Flesh. Bone.* The stump where it used to be gushed and gushed. *And if I don't stop there?* Then two pieces of the pronounced flesh of his chest vanished. *Slice. Stab. Saw.* Two silver-dollar sized wounds where his nipples used to be. *It's not stopping. His ears and those fat, squishy fucking cheeks*—I squeezed my eyes shut and looked in another direction.

"What's the matter, Dave? No comebacks this morning? Is it your period?"

"Huh? Oh, no, I'm just… Just still waking up. Long night. Give me an extra cup of that poison—I haven't had an ulcer in a while. And, for fuck's sake, Pop, you can't say shit like that."

"They can't fire me—I'm old!"

"Only one of those things is true, Pop," I said, as I grabbed my coffees and got the hell away from Dan and his knife.

I began forgetting things. What I'd done, where I'd been, who I'd talked to. Days blurred together without clear beginnings, middles, and ends. I couldn't keep track of tasks. They all became background static behind my constantly reeling mind. I didn't know if the forgetfulness was due to the lack of sleep, the increased alcohol consumption, or because I was simply losing my marbles.

One evening, after giving out medications to the kids with prescriptions, I left the keys to the medical office dangling from the lock. Then, inside the office, I left the keys to the medication locker out, too. Everything prescribed to any of these kids—all laid out for the taking. The boys could have found these and killed themselves, had they snuck out that night to steal food, which they did half of the damn time.

My supervisors reprimanded me the next day and wrote me up. They said they didn't have a choice. That it was gross negligence and the whole camp could have gotten into serious trouble. I felt devastated and overwhelmed with guilt. What if someone had gotten hurt? Overdosed on downers and died? And, to make things worse, I couldn't even remember going into the medical cabinet that night.

For months, I kept this reckless regimen. I increased the pace at work to distract myself. I flew from crisis to crisis at the camp, putting out whatever fires I could. I broke up fights, helped groups make dinner, made sure counselors got breaks for coffee or a smoke. Then I did it all over again. The harder I worked, the less I obsessed over nonsensical, violent, paranoid thoughts. It got harder to sleep, so I drank more at night. All day, I looked forward to some whiskey and, if I was lucky, a west coast basketball game still on TV. Then I got up at six to restart the whole cycle.

On a day off, I usually worked out for hours and hours. It distracted me, just like work did. It filled the spaces that intrusive thoughts otherwise occupied. If Annie and I weren't scheduled for time off together—or if the voices were too fucking loud for me to be around her—I ran, biked, and lifted weights until I was exhausted.

I considered talking to Annie about everything happening inside me. But what would I have even told her? That crazy images coursed through my head about hurting people? That I never slept and that I drank too much? That I might be losing my fucking mind? Annie was the best thing in my life, and I didn't want to scare her off.

I also thought about telling someone at work, like my boss. Or maybe one of the psychologists that worked at the camp. But I didn't want to concern them. They needed me. I was their workhorse—and I liked it. They already had enough people they couldn't rely on. I didn't want to be another wobbly wheel they had to replace.

And so, I went at it alone, riding the ups and downs of a condition I didn't yet know I had. On good days, I felt confident and bursted with energy. On bad days, violent images and shouting voices blitzed my mind. They could only be subdued with alcohol. I was trapped in a desperate and dreadful routine. But I thought I could at least keep it a secret and just maintain it. So I held on for dear life… until I couldn't.

Part Four

I

"Ohhh, won't you pleeease take me hooome!"

Fucking love this song. Fifty miles today. No problem. The pedals are pistons. Faster, faster, faster. Eleven days of work. I wasn't tired then and I'm not tired now. No sir. No chance. No how. Knowhow. Ha!

The sun. I can feel it. Energy into my skin and shooting out of my hands and feet.

I'm a machine.

Chili Peppers. Fuck yeah.

"... Making me lord of the moon!"

I am a motherfucking king. I'm flying over these hills. Maybe shopping later. Faster. Shoes, maybe. Harder. New Jordans. Yeah!

Trees, streams, trails. Magnificent. Faster.

Was that a frog? Damn. Flattened it. Flat frog. That flat frog had a family. That flat fucking frog had a fucking frog family that now must say farewell! Nice truck. F150 SVT, tuned. He's cruising.

"Yeeeaaaah, buddy! Get some!"

I'm alone in the universe. The stop sign has bullet holes. Why do people do that? So random. If a bullet hit me right now, I don't think it could slow me down.

That ride was easy. I need to do more. What's next? Jog to the track? I think I can run a five minute mile today. Always wanted to. Fuck it, why not?

Inhaling the meters in front of me. One lap down. I can go faster. Bounding. Soaring. Two laps. More, more, more. Give me more. Three laps. On pace. Let's fucking go. My heart and lungs are on fire. More gasoline. Let it fucking rip, Dave. Bang! Bang! Bang!

Four fifty eight!

"Oh, won't you flyyy hiiigh, freee biiird, yeah!"

Ready to call it a day. Easy jog home. I should really eat something. I wonder when they made these roads and what was here before. Nothing, I guess? Deer and sticks and—frogs!

Just another mile. Getting tired. Or, numb, maybe. Drifting, not running. Blood? When did I cut my leg?

Home. Things are quiet. Peaceful. It's dusk already. I think I might be able to finally fall asleep on my own tonight.

Couch. Bed is too far. Just lay down and sink.

II

The sun. It burns. I feel paralyzed, buried alive in this fucking couch. This feeling—dread or fear or fucking agony—it's crawling all over me. Is this real? Please, let this be a fucking nightmare. My heart is pounding. It's happening again. Shattered glass. Piercing shards in my head. I did this. I thought I made it go away yesterday. Ran it out of me. But I only made it worse. I've been out of control. I knew better. Why didn't I stop? Everything is wrong with me. Lazy, slow, stupid. Weak, insecure, useless. Not good enough. At anything. Not strong enough. Afraid. Broken piece of fucking shit, losing his fucking mind. Okay, get up. I need to move or the noise will get louder and louder. I think this is the worst I've ever felt in my whole life. What if I'm completely fucking helpless this time? I've been awake for three minutes. I'll never make it through the day. Each second passing hurts. Fuck me. Fuck fuck fuck. This could be the last thing I ever feel for the rest of my life. I need someone. Someone else's voice and not my own. Too much sun. People shouldn't see me like this but I can't be alone. What the fuck am I even going to say? Maybe they can just put their hand on my back and say something. Anything. And squeeze my shoulder. That would feel good. Help. Anything. Just not alone. My boss. I don't want him to know. But, fuck it, I don't care.

"Can we talk for a second?"

"Hey, Dave! Sure thing. How was your weekend?"

He thinks I'm fine. That I'm just checking in. Not fine. Not a check-in. Trying to speak. Just choking up. Tearing up. Fuck.

"Dave? Are you okay? What's going on? Hey man, talk to me."

I'm trying, but I can't. Just tears and my stupid, blubbering piece of shit fucking face.

"Wait here, Dave, I'm going to get Phil, the counselor."

Phil. The psychologist who works with the kids. I've thought about talking to him before. But I can't sit still and wait. I need to stand up. Move and walk and see something and do something. Anything but sit here and listen to the fucking voice in my head. I don't know what I'd say to Phil. I can barely think straight—how will I talk? Maybe alone is better. The empty campsite. No one's there right now. It's safe. I'm lost. Can't find it but I've been a hundred times. I'm losing my shit. The voice is getting louder and faster. I am gonna feel like this forever. The pain—it feels hot. It's burning inside my body. I have to get it out of me. I have to drain it. My knife. Always clipped to my belt. Heavy and cold. Swing it open. This is the right thing to do. Click. Let the pain flow out. In a stream of blood.

"Dave! Stop! Stop it now!"

It's Phil. How did he find me? He's grabbing me from behind. Pulling me to the ground. Twisting the knife out of my hand. I can't move. Can't even speak. The rest of my life—it'll be never-ending pain. Holding me tight. It's slowing down. Like last night. Getting quiet. Passing out, I think. Everything's fading away. Black.

How long was I out? In an empty room with a table and chairs. Phil's still here. And someone else. It's hard to keep my eyes open, so heavy. He wants me to take some pills. What are these? Who is he? Phil is saying it's fine. Okay whatever just take them. At least they brought me water. Where the fuck am I? Wait—a plastic bracelet on my wrist: Butler Psychiatric Hospital.

Chapter 3 - It Had a Name

"Good morning, David. How are you feeling today?"

How long have I been asleep? Is there any chance this is still just a long, awful nightmare? "Pretty out of it. What were those pills you gave me?"

"I'll tell you more about the medication. But first, I'd like to tell you what some of our observations and thoughts are at this stage. Would that be okay?"

I wasn't sure if I was ready to hear it, but I nodded.

"Well, based on what we've learned from speaking with you yesterday as well as with Phil, your symptoms indicate that you have likely been suffering from bipolar disorder."

Disorder. "What? What do you mean?"

"It is a condition characterized by alternating phases of depression and mania."

Illness. "Does it go away?"

"The symptoms can be reduced significantly and sometimes, nearly mitigated. There are very effective medications and treatment plans, which can include things like…"

It has a name. So I'm not the only one.

"David, did you hear me?"

"Sorry, what?"

"I asked if you'd be open to speaking with one of our psychologists today, to begin some counseling, and perhaps attend a group meeting."

"Okay. I think I could do that."

"Great, that is brave of you. The medicine we gave you was an antipsychotic. It helps to manage some of the more severe symptoms of bipolar and other disorders. We'd like to start you on some mood stabilizers and antidepressants that we believe could be very helpful."

Antipsychotic. Mood stabilizers. Bipolar. These were words I'd never contemplated—and they were breaking my world wide open. But at least it had a name. A name meant it was... a thing. A thing other people had, too. A name meant there could be help for it. Maybe this mania and depression that had tortured me for the last few years could go away.

But I asked myself, why *me*? Why did I get it? Did I give it to myself? Or was it always inside of me? If I gave it to myself, how was I so stupid as to not see it coming? If it was always there, like a dormant parasite, why wasn't I strong enough to keep it suppressed?

These questions were borne out of ignorance, not bias. I knew fuck-all about bipolar disorder. I understood that it was a mental illness, a scary one, and one I didn't think I'd ever have. Now that I did, it began to feel like a weakness. Something I needed help with—help I didn't want. And, certainly, medication I didn't want either.

They medicated me to the point of sedation. Pills and capsules in white, yellow, and green. Risperdal and Seroquel and Zyprexa. Then Abilify and Lamictal. Every couple of days, they added, subtracted, and mixed the doses. Even when I was awake, I was catatonic. Sleep and wakefulness blurred together. With those medications mixing with my blood and my brain, I wasn't myself—or what I thought was me. The desperate thoughts screaming through my head slowed and softened. But I didn't feel relief—I didn't feel *anything*. My energy—physical, emotional, all of it—was gone. But I didn't hurt as much. And I wasn't lying in a pool of blood somewhere in the woods.

I talked to a doctor every day. I couldn't keep track of the revolving cast of faces. Or maybe it was the same one every day, and I just kept forgetting. But they always asked the same litany of questions.

"How are you feeling today?"

"Okay."

"How are you feeling compared to yesterday?"

"A little better."

"Are the medications making symptoms improve?"

"It's hard to tell."

"Are the medications having any side effects?"

"Yes."

"What are they?"

"I still can't really tell if I'm awake or not…"

The rest of the wing consisted mostly of a big, open room strewn with pieces of furniture covered in blue vinyl, along with a few scattered coffee tables. Each table had some assortment of outdated magazines plopped on top, spread out in piles like old, dry, fallen leaves. Decorative, mostly. No one read them. There were also chess boards, checkers, and a few other games around the room. They all just sat in their boxes. The people there—they usually just sat, too.

Throughout the first few days, I wandered from couch to couch, trying to read a few pages of whatever magazines lay within arm's reach. It could have been a *Car & Driver, Sports Illustrated,* or even *Harper's*—it made no difference. I simply drifted in and out of sleep, waking periodically when a magazine landed in my lap.

On the third or fourth day, around mid-morning, Annie appeared. I couldn't figure out how she knew I was there. I thought no one but Phil had that information. Embarrassment burned in my stomach as soon as she saw me. She scooted up to me and wrapped me inside her arms. My own arms caught up and hugged her back after a few-second delay. I felt *almost* positive this was reality, but knew there was a chance I was dreaming. We only had an hour. Visiting times were short. *If you're still here after an hour, I guess it isn't real.*

"Hey." I didn't have a lot of words. I hoped she knew to expect that.

"Hey." She said just as little, instead clenching her arms even tighter around me.

I wanted to ask about work and the kids. But thinking about missing work made me feel guilty, so I avoided it. Instead, I half-assed an attempt at deflection. "Um, so how have you been?"

"I'm fine. Just thinking about you. I'm glad you're getting help here. I was so scared when Phil told me what happened."

"I know. I'm sorry I didn't talk to you more. I really didn't even know what was happening. I thought maybe I was just going crazy and—and I didn't know what to say."

"You're not. It's just a condition. You're going to get treatment and help just like you would for anything else. You're going to be fine."

"I hope so. I feel okay, now, I guess. But I'm just on all these fucking meds, so it's hard to tell. It's crazy—so many pills. I hate it."

"I know. But let them do their thing. They're doctors, right?"

"I think so. They've got those white coats on. Seems legit."

She laughed a bit. I felt the stiff creakiness of a face that hadn't smiled in days.

"Do you want me to call anyone for you?"

"No. Not now." I hadn't talked to my parents for a few months. My grandfather had just been diagnosed with brain cancer and didn't have long to live. Even if I wanted to tell them I was in the hospital, which I didn't, I couldn't bear to tell my mom just yet.

"You're going to be fine, and I'll be waiting for you," she said. Her eyes let me know she meant it.

Without sharing many words, we held onto each other for a long time, until visiting hours ended.

Chapter 4 - Justine

A big dry-erase board showed each day's group schedule. Some sessions covered cognitive behavioral therapy. Some focused on dual-diagnosis—mental illness and addiction. And some sessions were just labeled "open." For those, the doctor would encourage everyone to share. I suspected most of the people there weren't new. They knew what to say and how to navigate fluidly through this treatment. I cringed at the thought of coming back. To this place, or anywhere like it. *When I'm done, I won't ever see any of you again.*

The same three people talked most of the time during groups, pouring their stories into our laps. Amber stopped her medication again and thought she would hurt herself or her children. Becky's most recent depressive episode was so bad, all she could do was cry or sleep. I felt better knowing other people had some of the same thoughts as me.

But more than Amber or Becky or anyone else, Larry talked the most. I didn't mind at all. He entertained and distracted the rest of us from our own troubles. He obliterated awkward silences before they had a chance to fester. Whether he knew it or not, he filled in those empty spaces for all of us who didn't know what to say.

"They put some crack in those damn chicken nuggets, my God! But don't touch the pizza, or anything that fucking witch, Mitzi, makes. She's so fucking mean, man!"

Despite Larry and his endearing wackiness, I didn't feel connected to the others. Most of the faces there were long. The bodies moved slowly. The affliction I saw on them—it looked everlasting. The paranoia, the sadness, the confusion, whatever they had etched into their skin, it all looked permanent. I was there with them but needed to believe I was an aberration. Transitory, just passing through.

Justine was just like me, I thought. Different from the others. She had a life that seemed normal. A new boyfriend who she waxed dotingly about. A new job though not the one she wanted. Typical, twenty-something stuff. She talked a lot more than me. I didn't mind—it passed the time. Her words skipped and bounced around, stringing together random anecdotes. We made each other feel regular, sane, and safe. She reminded me of that popular girl in school who is nice to everyone, even the kids outside the cool crowd. *You don't look like you should be here. Do you think the same about me?*

She had a comforting, disarming smile and big, bright green eyes. She wore regular clothes every day, not the balloon-ish, blue hospital pants. She usually had on jeans that closely followed the lines of her legs and fitted sweaters that hugged the rest of her frame. Some days, though, she opted for her big, oversized Red Sox hoodie. Baggy sleeves shrouded her hands and a deep hood cast a shadow over her face. On those days, she was quieter.

Every morning and afternoon, most of the people from our wing took a walk outside around the hospital. Justine and I always walked together in the back, like the kids that sat in the rear of the bus. We walked the same path each day, never varying, even by a few steps. From the courtyard, a neat and tidy brick path took us around the white hospital complex. The path was lined with manicured red rose bushes, green hedges, and white flowering cherry trees.

"So, what are you doing when you leave? Are you gonna take some time off from work?" I asked her one day.

"I don't think so," she said. "Me and my boyfriend just got an apartment, and I have to cover half the rent. Plus I just started there and don't want to miss any more days."

Her talk of missing work gave me a sudden, sharp, guilty sting in my gut. "Right, yeah. So, do you like it there? Doing real estate stuff?"

"Yeah, I think so! It's just been admin work so far—you know, scanning and filing and all that. But I think I'll maybe go for my real estate license. You can make a lot more money once you get—"

She stopped when a thorn from a rose bush caught the floppy sleeve of the Red Sox sweatshirt, pulling it up toward her elbow. In that moment, I saw everything. A story of despair etched into her skin. She shoved her sleeve back down and stared straight ahead. Walking, but frozen. Until then I hadn't noticed that whether she donned tight sweaters or the big hoodie, she only wore long sleeves.

We were where we were supposed to be, after all. Justine was like me. And I was like her. Both ill. Both needing help. But not yet knowing how to receive it. I realized there were people out there like me. And some, like Justine, I could relate to. I could feel their pain. And them, mine.

She left a few days before me. It was harder without her. Our relatable small talk passed the time and felt reassuring. But in my solitude, I began to accept that I had an illness. I knew it was real and that I'd suffered for some time. I realized I wanted to leave the hospital with more than prescriptions. If nothing else, I knew I at least didn't ever want to come back. For that to happen, I needed to learn something, I reasoned. I didn't know what it was—or how I'd do it—but I figured the best place to start was by talking in group.

The next topic was dual-diagnosis, the coexistence of mental illness and substance abuse disorder. The psychologist leading the group welcomed everyone and recited her expectations. After a couple of weeks at Butler, it became clear how much drugs, alcohol, and mental illness intersected in the lives of people there. *My* life. Depression and bipolar swirled around freely with alcohol and coke and whatever else. Perfect dance partners. Or a perfect storm. I felt a burning in the pit of my stomach.

"Who would like to begin?"

I took a deep breath. "I'll start."

Everyone turned their heads quickly towards me, surprised to hear me and not Larry, Amber, or Becky. I didn't have anything thought out. I just let a medicated, blunt honesty lead the way. The medicine made it hard to string together my most thoughtful sentences, but it also made it easy to share them out loud. I was too numb for stage fright.

"About a year or two ago, I started having mood swings—or what I thought were mood swings. And then it turned into much more than that. I thought I was losing my mind. I'd be depressed for a week or two. And then—like, the opposite. Staying up all night, spending all my money—or maxing out my credit cards, actually, 'cause there was no money—getting fucked up a ton.

"I drink a lot. But since I started having these episodes, I drink more. To make the highs more… higher. Then, when I'm depressed, I drink to make the fucking voice in my head go away. And to stop thinking about hurting myself or other people. Weird, fucked-up images where I'm pushing people in front of a moving car or grabbing a knife and stabbing them. I obsess over this kind of shit. I'd never, ever, do any of it. But in the moment, it feels like something wants to take over my body and make me. Like a weird, demon animal might possess me. I can't—I can't even explain it.

"And then—I don't know. I guess it just got to be too much. I was really manic for a couple weeks and feeling so fucking great. One day I was running around all day, and I had all this energy and then—"

Tears started to form before I could push the last couple sentences out into the room.

"And then I woke up and I was just—broken. Completely fucking obliterated. It was suddenly the worst day of my life. I was, like, certain that I would never feel better. And I just didn't want to be alive anymore."

Everyone's eyes remained on me, but I couldn't quite finish and tell them what happened next, two weeks prior when Phil dragged me into his car and off to a hospital with white rooms. Everyone sat quietly. But I was okay with the silence. I didn't want feedback or a dialogue. And then the straight line between my friend Larry's sealed lips started to give way. *This should be good.*

"And *then* what happened?"

Before I could even crack a smile, the psychologist snapped, with a bit of force behind it, "Larry, please."

"I'm kidding!" He said, sporting a wild, delightful grin.

Her face relaxed a bit after I said, "It's okay. He's joking. I don't mind. Makes it easier."

"See?" Larry defended himself.

"But seriously," he started again, with a different face, "I tell myself this every day, and I have been for years. It's probably kept me alive. Listen to me—when you are spiraling into an episode and telling yourself that it is never going to get better, and that you'd be better off just fucking dead, shout over that voice in your head and scream to yourself: 'This episode will pass, like the ones before, and the ones yet to come. Even though it feels like it's going to be forever, it will always pass.'"

Some fog cleared for a moment when he said that. *It will always pass.* I loved the words, because in the middle of my episodes—when every invasive thought felt like a shard of glass digging and cutting deep into my fucking brain—the only thing that seemed certain in those moments was that it would never stop.

I left Butler with instructions, lists, and protocols. Four of these pills, two of these. And one of these (as needed). Call your doctor if *this* happens. Call 911 if *that* happens. Schedule a monthly check-in with a psychiatrist. Find a therapist. Don't mix your medications with drugs or alcohol or you may trigger episodes.

Over the course of two weeks, I'd snapped out of the idea that I was there by accident. I planned on taking my pills—a hearty blend of mood stabilizers, antidepressants, and antipsychotics—because I never wanted to relive that day. I even planned to make an appointment to talk to Phil every week. But I still thought that I was, somehow, different from the other people. The permanence of it—I didn't think it applied to me. I figured I could get back to life as I knew it if I just took my doses every morning. I had no plans of identifying myself as someone with bipolar. I had the misguided notion that if I was strong, I could somehow *beat* it.

A miscalculation that almost killed me.

Chapter 5 - Don't Operate Heavy Machinery

When I got back to the whirlwind of my daily work, I avoided telling anyone that didn't need to know. Annie knew. Phil, who'd saved my fucking life, of course knew. My boss, whose office I'd broken down in, had at least a clue. And I told Will and Alex, my two best friends, who eventually would see, hear, and feel it. Other than that, the only other souls I cared to share this secret with were the anonymous Duane Reade pharmacists who'd fill my 'scripts.

As far as everyone else at work was concerned, I'd gotten real sick with the flu. Everyone bought the story because I'd never let them see what was really happening inside me. But as I reintegrated into work, I found it hard to be my old self. The new regimen of medications left me staggered. Before Butler, energy pumped through me like an electric current. Afterward, that crisp electricity had been replaced with thick, numb lethargy. I mostly just wanted to sleep. If I couldn't sleep, I wanted to lie down. If I couldn't lie down—well, then I would sit my ass down on a rock and let my head droop into my chest.

In the first few weeks, I felt too tired to even be concerned about the kids. I couldn't remember what issues they had been dealing with when I left. And I didn't really care. Counseling them became a chore. It felt like another thing keeping me from my sleep. Before I left, when kids had meltdowns, got aggressive, or ran away from the group, I lit up and sprang into action. When Eric ran into the woods, trying to find the damn highway, I would've run ten times as far after him. But after Butler, between one task and the next, sometimes I'd find a hiding place, lie down, and give in to the Zyprexa until my radio started blaring at me.

I tried going for a run on my first weekend off. I didn't feel like it—at all—but I hadn't worked out in a couple weeks. I had a quick four-mile course that I'd perfectly mapped out and done dozens of times. I had almost gotten down to twenty-four minutes, a six-minute-mile pace. Before I landed in the hospital, I remember being certain I would get it on the next try. I expected to be a bit slower, but not like this. It felt like I was running in combat boots. I finished in thirty-one minutes. Just weeks prior, that was a warm-up pace. But my body wasn't mine anymore.

My mind wasn't my own, either. I couldn't concentrate on tasks. One day, after driving one of the kids to a meeting with his parole officer, I got out of the car but left it in *drive*. I stumbled along after it, trying to hop back in and get to the brakes. But it had already picked up too much speed. It didn't stop until the front bumper lodged itself around a thick tree trunk. That was the last time I got assigned anything requiring a vehicle.

My supervisors and colleagues started asking less of me. They knew something was amiss and stopped relying on me as often to watch their groups or join on their day trips. I felt guilty that I couldn't give them as much as I used to. I wanted to explain. I wanted to let them know I just needed time to adapt to this new treatment and medication. But I kept all of it private.

I felt relieved to be around Annie again, but as safe as I was in her arms, I was equally exposed. I thought it might be easier to drift away rather than be so vulnerable. But I couldn't—she wouldn't let me. She thought the good stuff was still there. The enthusiasm to help these kids. The energy to run and jump and play. The gusto to take off for a ski trip at five a.m. with a girl I'd just met, hungover but charged with Dunkin' and spontaneity.

When we first started dating, we went out every weekend, whatever the season. We explored New England. Biking, skiing, hitting the beach—whatever we could think of. When we were snowed in, we made scavenger hunts for each other, hiding favorite DVDs and candy around the house. But after Butler, we didn't bike in the summer and fall. We didn't do scavenger hunts when we were snowed in. My creativity had been suffocated. Instead, we watched movies, ate, and slept a lot. Annie pretended to sleep next to me when I napped in the middle of the day. I knew she got up once she heard me snoring.

And when I was trapped inside my mind, unable to even settle into a dumb movie, we didn't do anything at all.

"I don't know if you should wait for me."

"It's okay, we can just sit here. I don't mind."

"No, I mean, like…" I took a deep breath and then finished. "Maybe you should move on. I don't know what's left for you to wait for."

"Stop it. Everything I love about you is still here. I feel it. Just give it some time. I'll wait, for as long as it takes."

After a few weeks, my system finally acclimated to the drugs. For the last couple of months of my time at the camp, I was stable. I didn't have the motor I did before getting hospitalized, but I didn't need to take quick naps on piles of dirt.

They held a celebration every time a counselor completed their two years. That's how rarely it happened—it needed a special fucking event. They wanted both me and Annie to stay longer, of course. But I was done. I needed that chapter to be over. Every step I took at the camp reminded me of something that hurt—the worst invasive, manic, and suicidal thoughts. I'd be happy to never even see Rhode Island again.

With all the kids and counselors and staff gathered in the dining hall, the camp director kicked it off. "I remember my phone screen with David. I was a little concerned that this city kid from California might not have what it takes to work here. But when he said he went to college in New Hampshire, I figured he wouldn't complain about the cold and that he probably knew how to start a campfire."

I played along. "Oh, come on, man, I don't like where this is going…"

"But when I picked his butt up at the airport in the middle of winter, and the guy was standing in the snow wearing a hoodie and some Air Jordans, I had serious concerns."

The joke got some good laughs. I had famously forgotten to bring a winter jacket with me back to the East Coast. I only had my black Cal State Long Beach hoodie—the same one Juan wore when the cops took him back to jail—to combat the rain and snow. They thought it made an endearing anecdote about my West Coast predilections. They didn't know I'd left my coat behind because I could barely put one foot in front of the other, much less put a proper suitcase together.

"But while he didn't know how to make a fire, he turned into one of the best counselors we've ever had." Then he turned towards me. "The hard work, the commitment you've shown—it's truly the example we want all counselors to follow. We wish you were staying, but we know you'll be an incredible addition to the next team you're a part of."

The kids and the other counselors clapped, then stood up. But it didn't feel real. I felt embarrassed that I hadn't finished stronger. That I'd needed to go on medication. That the medication made me spend more time sleeping and less time counseling. One of the best counselors they've ever had? No chance.

They're clapping for… an imposter.

Part Five

Chapter 1 - California Love

After Rhode Island, Annie and I decided to move to San Francisco. We had a cluster of friends there—mostly college friends who'd made their way west. My family also lived nearby, scattered throughout Oakland and Berkeley. We got an apartment in the Marina district. The main drag looked like a university frat row on steroids. Every weekend, drunk twenty-somethings, stuck between college and real life, spilled in and out of the dozens of bars lining the streets.

I was still trying to take the doctors' advice and not drink *too* much. So, moving to the Marina was a risky choice for me. The bars sat so close to our apartment that we could hear them from our couch. It was a tempting, seductive lure that I was better off without. On the other hand, we lived near friends.

After a few weeks of blasting out resumes and begging whoever I could for introductions, I landed a job in real estate with an excellent boss and mentor. He and his partners brought me into their firm, hoping they had landed a young, smart, and ambitious kid ready to break into the commercial real estate game. And that's who they got, for a time.

Annie took another job in social work. Ceaselessly compassionate, she was willing to stay in the difficult line of work, this time shifting her focus from kids in juvenile justice to kids in foster care. I wanted to get into business and hopefully support some long-term financial growth. But I didn't want to stop working with kids, so I tutored on the side. It made me feel good and gave us a little extra cash while I tried to get the real estate job underway.

Before long, I turned the tutoring side-hustle into a part-time business venture with another tutor I met, who'd just formed a company and was looking for a partner. We put together a team of a dozen part-time tutors that taught kids all over the Bay Area. I worked about sixty or seventy hours each week. During normal office hours, I sought out new clients and new transactions for our real estate firm. At night and on weekends, I worked on the tutoring business and grew our little brand.

We were off to a great start. I worked hard and didn't drink much. Annie was happy in her new job. I also made sure to hit the ground running with my treatment. With a few weeks before my new health insurance kicked in, I ran out of my meds. Not wanting to interrupt the medication, I went to refill my prescriptions at retail price. The pharmacist rang up my full menu of goodies: Lamictal, the mood-stabilizer; Zoloft, the anti-depressant; and Risperdal, the break-glass-in-case-of-emergency anti-psychotic. I knew it would be expensive… but not seven hundred dollars.

"Sorry, sir. Your card didn't go through."

"Oh, really? Shit. Okay, hang on a second. I'll be right back."

I slinked into one of the aisles to avoid any embarrassing eavesdropping while I made a phone call.

"Hey, babe. Umm… you got any space on your credit card? I'm in a bit of a pickle over here at Walgreens."

Chapter 2 - The Doctor Will See You Now

I didn't want to keep seeing a doctor. But I needed my prescriptions, so I'd have to whether I liked it or not. I was nervous heading into my first appointment with Dr. Ewing. I'd just started to feel comfortable with the meds—I didn't want him to tinker with them. The lethargy had decreased. Some of my old energy had come back, but without as much of the mania, depression, and obsessive thoughts.

But I also just didn't want to have to tell the story all over again. I didn't want to share with a stranger the grim details of my mood swings, invasive thoughts, heavy drinking, and my stint at Butler Psychiatric Hospital. I didn't want a new expert in my ear, telling me the who, what, where, when, why, and how of my treatment.

But besides the intake paperwork, the appointment with Dr. Ewing was quick. The session lasted only half an hour, and I spent the first ten minutes in his foyer waiting for him to call me in.

"Hi, I'm Doctor Ewing," he said once I got inside. He extended his hand.

A handshake felt a little transactional for a psychiatry appointment, but I didn't mind. "I'm David. Nice to meet you."

I sat on the small couch he had for patients, and he plopped down on a contraption that could only be described as a medicine ball with wheels. With quite perfect posture, he looked at me, quizzically, from his unique perch.

Oh, great, you're going to make me do all the talking? "So, I guess I should just give you a little bit of background?"

"Yes, please do." He felt chilly and awkward to me. Like an alien doing its best impersonation of a human mental health practitioner.

I gave him the skinny—my first episode, my self-medicating in Rhode Island, and my time at Butler. I did, however, leave out the part where Phil stopped me from cutting my wrist in the middle of the woods. I did, however, share my lingering concerns about the meds making me heavier and slower. It was a dubious attempt to keep him from recommending even more of it.

He homed in on the alcohol, not my mile times, "Are you still drinking now?"

"Not as much as before." It wasn't a lie. But for some reason I still felt the tinge of guilt that usually hit after bullshit left my mouth.

"I see. I would stress the importance of minimizing drug and alcohol use. They can trigger manic or depressive episodes. It's also not good to mix alcohol with some of the medication you're taking, particularly the—"

Okay, I get it. I didn't want to hear the rest. I'd heard that a half dozen times already. "I'll keep that in mind."

After a few months, I got a bit too comfortable and lost focus on treatment. I could so quickly forget how far I'd come, just from missing the feeling of being high. I skipped my pills every few days, seeking out the little buzz of energy that came from lifting the covers off my flat, numbed, medicated self. And, sure enough, if I did feel hints of mania and depression, I let alcohol quickly close up the wound.

Just a little bit at first. A few sips at night to relax and slow down the sharp, pointy thoughts that zigzagged around my mind. A few more on the weekends, to cut loose with friends. Annie often came out with me. We'd drink a bit together with my old friends, and her new ones. But when she wasn't out with me, I drank more in the absence of her mindful eye. If she said she was tired and wanted to stay in, I lamented outwardly. But inside, I was not disappointed.

Chapter 3 - Hat Trick

Drinking came so easily in the city. I was around more friends, more parties, and more bars. In Rhode Island, I often had to drink by myself and plan when and where to get my booze. They didn't put the camp for juvenile offenders around the corner from any liquor stores. But in San Francisco, I always had access, and I always had company.

I drank most often with Alex and James. Alex had been back in the Bay Area since college, teaching and coaching lacrosse at his old middle school. He waited with arms wide open when I arrived. We still had the same appetite for weightlifting, Guns N' Roses, and a cool thirty-pack of Bud Light. Or a warm one, to be sure.

James had become a close friend at Dartmouth. He was a recruit on the rowing team, and he kicked my ass all throughout freshman year. Not quite the consummate masochist like the rest of the rowing cohort, he did an obligatory year and then moved on. He was a different kind of drinking partner than Alex. He liked to socialize and take part in the San Francisco nightlife without blacking it out of existence. As long as I got fucked up, though, I didn't really care if I was at a nice bar with James or in a basement with Alex.

In addition to the old crew, I gathered up a list of new, interchangeable drinking partners. First, I found Blake. I could call him any night of the week, even after the bars closed, and he'd be up for getting lit. The business partner I found for the tutoring company also had a penchant for drinking. At our first meeting, we'd gotten hammered at a sushi restaurant as we excitedly mapped out our plans on soy sauce-stained napkins.

Blake ended up getting hooked on Vicodin. He stayed with us for a couple weeks when his girlfriend kicked him out. Then Annie kicked him out after he used our money to buy more pills. I didn't see Blake for years after that. Shortly after he left our place, he landed in rehab.

My tutoring partner's drinking led to pills, too. But he didn't stop there. Eventually he started shooting up heroin. I found out after stumbling upon late night ATM withdrawals all over San Francisco from our business checking account. The late-night debits sewed the early demise of our partnership.

The most seductive new drinking partner, though, was Zach. He was an angry drunk, always looking for fights when we walked around the city streets together. Something about his aggression enticed me. I always backed him up and usually egged him on. And, eventually, I started seeking out little tastes of it right along with him.

One night, we came up on about five guys around two in the morning, after the bars had closed. There were a few girls with them. As the distance closed between us, we saw the sidewalk clearly didn't hold enough room for both groups.

"Let's make them get out of the way," he said, "and see what they do."

As we crossed paths, we each made sure to bump shoulders with the guys, daring them to push back. What I didn't see, though, was Zach whispering something to one of the girls. I didn't hear it, but they sure did.

"Fuck you, asshole!" said one of the girls.

"What's your problem, bro?" An angry friend rushed to her defense, pushing Zach.

"We aren't your fucking bros," I said as I darted in front of Zach and quickly snapped my arms straight, right into the guy's chest. He stumbled backward and stayed there while he looked at me. They vastly outnumbered us. I intensified my stare, knowing that if we conveyed any fear, we would probably get our asses kicked.

"Let's get the fuck out of here," the guy said, "these assholes are fucked up."

I felt disgusted with myself the next morning. I knew that wasn't who I was, yet I continued to do it, especially if I was with someone like Zach. It felt like something dormant inside—an angry, fanged animal—wrested control from me. The guilt always remained after that behavior, but it became more subdued as the drunken aggression got more normal. I didn't know what had changed in me, or where the animal came from. I thought maybe it was the prescriptions. Before I was diagnosed and taking medication, I never became a hostile drunk like that. I was a lot of things—horny, self-destructive, goofy, guilt-ridden, incontinent—but never a menace to others. But now, after enough drinks, a switch flipped. And because I was drinking more, the animal saw more and more daylight.

Sure enough, Zach eventually went to rehab, too. It was a rehab hat trick. Three of the people I'd spent the most time with were all admitted before they were thirty. All smart college grads with promising starts to their careers. But all loaded to the brink with booze and drugs.

As I drank more and more with these new and old accomplices, I spent less time with Annie. Of course, I didn't love her any less. But I loved alcohol, too, and had to slide her over a bit to make more room for both. She knew I drank, but she didn't know how much. I often told her I was going to see a movie with Alex, but we would go out drinking instead. Or that James and I were just going to grab dinner, but we'd end up in a nearby bar. I convinced myself I was some sort of MacGyver when it came to concealing the smell of alcohol on my breath or sneaking a flask around. Fat chance.

The more I drank with others, the more I could try to make it seem normal to Annie and to myself. But for all the booze I drank with Alex, James, Blake, or Zach, I depended on none of these friends to enable my habit as much as Will. Wherever he was in the world, Will and I were unwavering, inseparable drinking partners.

Chapter 4 - Goodnight, Sweet Prince

Will and I had become best friends during my sophomore year on the rowing team. We approached the sport the same way—with abandon. Everyone on our crew team got after it. It was typical for the whole squad to lie out on the floor of our boathouse after every practice. But while everyone was frantically catching their breath, Will and I were often throwing up. Our teammates chased excellence. But Will and I ran from guilt—an even stronger motivator. Will had his own bouts with depression and mood swings. He'd later come to reconcile with them, like I would. When we were in college, we didn't know where those emotions came from, what they were called, or how to talk about them. So, whether the reasons were spoken or not, we shared a deep empathy and comfort with one another.

After college, the reckless training subsided. It gave way to work schedules and waning motivation to stay in shape. But the reckless drinking persisted. He took a job in Chicago, but that didn't stop us. We logged on to Skype and put back our respective bottles of whiskey while we jabbered, played online Scrabble, or watched a DVD in sync. We kept Skype on, even as our conversation subsided and we faded to sleep, finding comfort in the sight of a drink in one another's hands until the very end. We were together, no matter how far apart.

Every couple of months, we visited each other and binged for a weekend. We did the same stuff we did on Skype, just more of it, and with a lot more alcohol. A Scrabble board, cigarettes for Will, dipping tobacco for me, and a few DVDs we'd watched dozens of times. That was all we needed. Sometimes we went to the bars, but only if we ran out of alcohol or other friends made us.

We drank the cheap whiskey. The stuff that comes in plastic bottles—Canadian Mist, Royal Mist, or some other kind of generic "Mist." We drank so much liquor we had to quite seriously consider the cost of buying Jack Daniels or Seagram's, let alone Maker's Mark. We could get two 1.75L handles for under thirty bucks, as long as we just stuck to one of the "Mists."

Before leaving for my next winter sojourn in Chicago, I went for a run. Maybe five miles or so. I hadn't stayed in good shape, but I ran hard, knowing I would get obliterated for the next three days. Like crew practice back in school, the exercise made me feel less guilty about a previous, or impending, bender. Will and I planned to get in a run or two. Wishful thinking, perhaps.

Will picked me up from O'Hare on a Friday evening. After a few minutes of breathing in the biting December air mixed with exhaust from shuttle buses, I saw his head poke out of his car window, his eyes wide and bright and joyful.

"My sweet prince!" He shouted the nickname we shared, which dated back to sophomore year of college. The moniker had stayed intact, though its origin was long forgotten.

I sloshed my way through the dark, muddy snow outside arrivals at O'Hare. "It was sixty-eight and sunny back home, you know?"

"Hey, man, it's your turn to fly. Fair is fair," he said, as I hurriedly tossed my bag in the back and hopped into shotgun. "We can't all live in San Francisco drinking kombucha all day."

"Okay. But the 'booch is fantastic."

On the way to his apartment, we stopped at Dominick's Supermarket to get alcohol, tobacco, and a meal. The cashier's eyes widened as our selections slid down the conveyor belt: two handles of Royal Mist whiskey and a DiGiorno's Supreme pizza, thick crust.

"Anything else?" she asked, chuckling at us.

"Oh, um, also can I get a pack of Camel Lights?" Will asked.

I gave him a nudge.

"Sorry, and a tin of mint Skoal."

"Yum," she offered.

With our wares in hand, we felt free and liberated. We had an entire weekend to drink ourselves silly. On the chilly walk back to his apartment, we were giddy, like children at the tippy top of a roller coaster ride, brimming with visceral excitement in anticipation of the first plunge.

As soon as we got back to his apartment, we opened the big bottle and poured. The fifteen-dollar swill felt as invigorating as some fine single malt—or close enough. As always, the first sip tasted like the thing missing from my body. I closed my eyes and took a deep breath, letting the alcohol fill the empty little crevices in me. After our first drink, Will brought out the Scrabble board.

"I flew all the way out here, and the first thing we do is play Scrabble?"

"Better believe it. Take a drink after any thirty-point move?"

"Ummm... Let's make it twenty-five."

We were both pretty good. We liked to believe it was because of our English B.A. degrees from Dartmouth. But it was because we played all the fucking time. As we ran out of asinine anecdotes and multisyllabic Scrabble plays, we shifted our gaze to the background movie, *Heat,* just in time for Pacino and De Niro to face off outside the airport. Our first handle of whiskey had expired, as did we. We melted into unconsciousness, just as the sun cracked through the window blinds.

"Fuck!" I said, after waking up in the early afternoon.

"Yeah. We drank the whole bottle," he said, coughing, "and I think I finished that whole pack of Camels. Yuck."

"No, I mean we slept so late. It's almost dark!" The sun had almost set over the awesome Chicago skyline, before I even caught a glimpse of it.

"As much as you hate it, we have to sleep at some point this weekend, too."

"Okay, well, let's just get up and make some afternoon-coffee. What about our run?"

"It's not happening. It was never happening."

"Yeah, I know." I was starting to get out of shape, big time. A surge of guilt shot through me, regretting the wasted hours we could have spent together, jogging or otherwise.

"Don't forget, we've got that dinner with Greg and Keith."

I *had* forgotten. We had agreed to have dinner with a couple of guys from Dartmouth who lived in the area. They weren't my favorites. It felt obligatory. Punitive, even. When Will made the mistake of telling them I was coming to town, they promptly invited themselves to hang out with us.

It was evening when we left the apartment for the first time that day. I popped a small handful of medication—the ones I forgot to take the night before *and* the ones I was supposed to take in the morning that I'd just slept through. The pills made me nauseous on an empty stomach, but we were about to get some Chicago deep-dish.

We squirmed our way through small talk like fidgety students sitting through a boring class. As tasty as it was, deep-dish was a bad choice if our aim was to keep dinner brief. It took damn near ninety minutes to get our food on a packed Saturday night at Lou Malnati's.

"It's going great at Lehman. We've had a huge quarter. It's gonna be a big year." Keith's voice was too loud for me to tune out the boring conversation about work. "And—the best part—I made vice-president."

"Yeah, cool, but isn't *everyone* at investment banks a vice-president? I feel like that's on every business card," I said, with a lonely smirk.

I thought I resented them for their all-work-and-no-play attitude. But I actually just resented that they were doing better than I was. Their ambition, aptitude, and education propelled them forward. Meanwhile, after a strong start at my real estate firm and an exciting, though brief, small business venture, I'd fallen behind. I did enough to get by, but not much more. I'd spent too many of my workdays swimming in and out of hangovers. I came in late and bleary-eyed from the night before or left early to catch friends at a happy hour.

Instead of feeling free and liberated, like the night before, I felt guilty and trapped. Will did a better job of acting interested. Maybe he actually was—but I don't think he knew what derivatives were, either. He was just more polite than me. As Keith and Greg jabbered on, I tuned them back out and once again considered the pros and cons of deep-dish.

After dinner, I wanted to get lit. Bad. I was in a shitty mood after hearing about derivatives and fucking mortgage-backed securities. We ditched those guys and resumed drinking, only the two of us, like I wanted. We drank late into the night, letting alcohol rewind time as we reminisced about crew races won and pretty girls lost. As the night crested its way towards last-call, I felt a flood of deep, overwhelming love for my best friend and most devout drinking partner. *If only this could be the way it was, always.* Alcohol has a way of blissfully stopping time, but just for the ones drinking.

Will couldn't walk home on his own after the bars emptied out. I propped him up as we stumbled in what I hoped was the right direction. I found Will's building after some meandering. I dug his keys out of his pocket and corralled him through the lobby and into the elevator. As soon as I opened the door to his apartment, he crashed to the ground. I dragged him to his bed and laid him down. I wished he was still awake with me, but he looked peaceful. *Goodnight, Sweet Prince.*

He gave me a ride to the airport early the next morning. We were still foggy—or still drunk. As we turned onto the main thoroughfare, I finally saw it —Lake Michigan. It looked like the damn ocean. The opposite shore was completely out of view, well beyond the horizon. I hadn't even seen it once, because we'd been too wasted to get up while the sun was still out. I quickly closed my eyes.

Chapter 5 - No Balls, No Babies

Annie offered to pick me up at SFO. I certainly didn't want to take the train—not with its tight, crowded spaces and recirculated air—but I didn't want to see her yet. Rather, I didn't want *her* to see *me* yet. I looked like I'd been binging all weekend, of course. Probably smelled like it, too, despite a hurried shower at Will's before hustling to the airport. I told her I'd take the subway and see her at home.

I hadn't thought about work since the week before, and I couldn't remember what was scheduled for the next day. This had become typical—weekends so destructive that I couldn't even pick up Monday where I'd left off. I regressed each week, working five days, then going backwards for two.

After a deep breath, I checked my calendar on the subway train. *Shit! What was I thinking, scheduling this for tomorrow?* I had a full day of tours with a client to look at almost a dozen retail sites. His flight from Los Angeles was scheduled to land at 6:30 a.m., a couple hours south in San Jose. I said I'd be there to pick him up. The worst part? I couldn't fucking stand this guy. His name was Dennis Dixon, but he preferred to go by "Double-D." In addition to stupid nicknames, he also had a penchant for stupid catch phrases. *Winner winner chicken dinner. Hasta la vista, baby.* And his favorite: *No balls, no babies.* Cringeworthy stuff.

Annie was in bed when I finally got home. I slept on the couch, not wanting to wake her or make her suffer with me when my alarm went off at 4:30 a.m. A few short hours later, when my phone started blaring in my ear, I laid still, hoping I was dreaming. *Maybe I'm still in Chicago with Will, with one more day of drinking and escape in front of me?* Nope. I made coffee straightaway, before even brushing my teeth. It was acidic and sour when it hit my stomach.

"Hey, babe," Annie said, rubbing her eyes. "Why are you up so early?" Her voice startled me more than the sour coffee.

"Sorry, sweetie, I didn't mean to wake you." She looked adorable, half-awake with her hair all over the place. I felt guilty the moment I saw her. "I've got to pick up this client in San Jose in a couple hours."

"Why did you schedule that for this morning?"

"Fantastic question."

"Well, good job waking up on time, I guess. Just drive safe, okay?"

"I will. I made some coffee."

"Gross, babe, that looks awful," she said as she peered into the pitch black cup. "You really don't know how to make coffee."

I drifted asleep on the road a few times, waking up when the bumps in between lanes jolted my Mazda. I'd finished my coffee, so I pulled over to get a Red Bull. A disgusting combination, but I needed both to get there without any more dangerous, high-speed catnaps.

I arrived a little early and parked in the cell phone lot, ecstatic to close my eyes for even a few extra minutes. I reclined my seat a few notches and fantasized. *Maybe his plane had a malfunction? Not like, crashed. Fuck me, I'm an asshole. But, yeah, maybe something small and it couldn't take off?* No such luck. My phone started chirping with his text messages. Double-D had arrived.

I'd come woefully unprepared for the site visits. While on the subway the night before, I'd frantically sent out emails begging other brokers for last-minute tours of their locations. Some, bless their hearts, had actually agreed despite the egregiously short notice. For the rest, we'd have to look through the window. I'd lie and say the rest had canceled or called in sick.

He flopped his big, overweight body down in the passenger seat. I felt the car lurch to the right and silently apologized to my Mazda.

"Hey, man!" he hollered into my ears, which already rang.

"Double-D in the house!" *Fake it till you make it, Dave.*

"Where are we headed? You ready to get this show on the road?"

Couldn't be less ready. "Yes, sir! Let's do it."

He started yapping as soon as we headed up to San Francisco. Weather. Girls. Football. After a while, I couldn't hear him anymore. Instead, I heard my head pounding like a drum and my stomach trying to sort out the coffee, Red Bull, and lingering deep dish pizza. I wasn't listening—but I pretended, eking out a chuckle whenever it seemed like the right moment.

How can I treat work like this? I can't even string together a couple thoughtful sentences. How am I going to talk about prices per square foot, capital improvement allowances, or lease terms? This guy sucks, but I need the money. It would be a wasted day. Another one. Just like many, many others.

I trudged through San Francisco, counting down tour stops like a restless kid counting down minutes until the school bell rang out. I needed to sleep. I needed to eat something nourishing. And I needed peace and quiet from streetcar brakes groaning, horns honking, and, most of all, Double-D.

Finally, after the tenth tour, the day crawled to its end. Thankfully, he took a cab to the airport. All that was left was a wrap-up meeting.

I asked, "So which site works best? Which are we making an offer on?" *Let's cut to the chase, please.*

"Definitely Market Street. That's the winner."

"Yeah, the foot traffic is unbeatable. Let's talk offer terms—what are you thinking?" *Okay, now don't blow it, Dennis.*

"Let's hit 'em with eighty percent of asking price, and a couple hundred thousand bucks in improvements to the space."

Jesus. The Art of the Deal, by Double D. "Uh—Dennis, we can't go so low. We'll just piss them with an offer like that."

"Come on, man! No balls, no babies! Am I right?"

"Whatever you say. I'll write it up," I relented, vastly too tired to argue.

I need to get my shit together. The thought darted through my mind every damn day. I wondered if the partners at the firm realized yet that they'd overestimated my potential. I'd convinced myself I could still play hard if I just worked harder, too. I thought I could make up for a lost day by just working late the next night. But I could never catch up faster than I fell behind.

Worse, still, I tricked myself into thinking I actually *was* functioning at my potential, or close enough to it. I chalked up wasted workdays, like the one I spent with Double-D, to bad timing, bad scheduling, or bad fortune, instead of holding myself to account. It's insidious, the way my addicted mind could lie and distort.

Sometimes, it was, *Hey, just because you're running late and fighting a hangover doesn't mean you can't get just as much done.* And then, maybe, *Don't worry, you wouldn't be doing any better at work if you weren't drinking and getting fucked up all the time.* Or, perhaps the most subversive deception: *Other people just can't handle work and drinking like you can. They're missing out. Losers.* But of course, I couldn't get as much done. Of course, I could have done better work. And, of course, the only person missing out was me.

I let myself believe a reckless drinking habit wouldn't slow me down on the career front. It was all bullshit, about as reasonable as expecting to run my best race while carrying a sixty-pound stone under one arm. How could reckless drinking *not* have been an obstacle in the pursuit of a profession? But that's the evil genius of addiction. You can talk yourself into anything to get your fix.

Part Six

Chapter 1 - Season's Greetings

I was first to arrive at my grandparents' house for Christmas dinner. Annie had gone to Florida to spend the holiday with her brother. I accidentally showed up an hour early after too hastily reading the invitation. They were at their neighbors', having a glass of wine. Alone in their home, I remembered my childhood summers.

Just like when I was little, it still felt like I was in a museum. Awards, souvenirs, medals. And hundreds of books covering the A to Z of American history: the Civil War, the Industrial Revolution, famous generals, and the presidents. The all-stars, of course, like Washington, Lincoln, and Roosevelt. But they even had a book about Gerald Ford, just in case any of their guests were overcome with interest in the thirty-eighth president.

But my ephemeral enjoyment dissolved when I saw the mound of holiday cards on their kitchen countertop. *Look at the shiny faces on all these people. Their skin pulled tight from an hour of smiling for extended photo shoots. My face is never shiny. Not this time of year.* Christmas always brought me back to memories of my own family's many meltdowns. They followed me all year, lurking, ready to resurface every fucking December.

At that moment, I recalled my dad drinking on the way to dinner at the Persian restaurant we went to every Christmas Eve. At our table, things would seem okay, at first. An onlooking diner or waiter might even think we were a normal family having a lovely, splendid

Christmas Eve. But they couldn't see the tight undercurrent of dread running through me, my sisters, and my mom.

The smallest of things triggered him. Less than small. If my sister or I took too much bread at the table. *Greedy.* If one of us forgot to say thank you for passing a dish. *Ungrateful.* If we were too eager for Christmas presents the next morning. *Spoiled rotten.* Heads around us turned when his fists slammed down on the table.

On the way home, anger would continue bursting out of his narrow eyes, taut lips, and clenched fingers. He jerked the steering wheel and punched the gas pedal while my sisters and I sat frozen in the back seat. This, all from the lightest, feathery touch to a short temper imbued with alcohol.

And so, all those years later, that's what I saw when I looked at the pile of holiday cards. I needed to drink. Fortunately, finding alcohol at my grandparents' house was as easy as finding a biography of George Washington. Or Gerald Ford, apparently. I prepared to see the gaggle of extended family by rounding up five little bottles of single-serve liquor. They were all compliments of various airlines, hotels, and casinos, saved for later use by two famously thrifty grandparents.

The first drink. A novelty bottle of Jack Daniels. *The smell. I love it. A deep inhale. Pins and needles from my lungs to my fingertips.* The first sip of alcohol washed me in relief.

Second drink. A tiny green bottle of Jägermeister. *Jägermeister... An odd choice for them. But free.* I never loved the taste of Jägermeister, but right then it was just fine. My chest and arms warmed. My eyes slowly closed.

Third drink. A shot of Absolut Vodka. *Clear, crisp, and clean.* After I finished the little bottle, I breathed a few deep, resounding breaths.

Fourth drink. An ounce and a half of Hendrick's Gin. *Alcohol and blood, mixing together, becoming singular.* My throat was almost numb. The gin went down so smoothly and easily.

Fifth drink. Maker's Mark. *Best for last.* After the last drop hit the back of my throat, I sat down in my grandfather's recliner and leaned back. I felt peace, calm, and silence for the rest of my time alone.

When I heard the car doors closing and chatter outside, I quickly put the little bottles in the recycling bin and buried them good. I'd drift through the next few hours like I wasn't really there. I'd be my own body double, filling in for an anxious and dejected self. I'd make this Christmas sufferable, after all. *Maybe I can even smile enough for a holiday card.*

"Aunt Debra! How are you? So good to see you!" I said, standing inches from the doorway when she swung it open.

"Oh! Wow, you startled me. Merry Christmas, David. I'm going to go set down the dessert I brought."

My cousin stood next in line, after my aunt slinked by. "Molly! My favorite cousin! Bring it in for a hug!"

"Jeez, settle down, man. We just got here. We have a long night ahead of us, and I haven't had any wine yet. Wait—have you?"

"Mom! Dad! I beat you guys here! Let me get those for you." I ignored Molly's inquiry and took a few plates of side dishes from my parents.

It was fun for an hour or two. I played a character. Smiles and sweaters and cheers and hugs. But I could only subdue the pain and angst lingering from years ago for so long. I was still hurt on the inside. The liquor dug in and turned that pain outward. By the time we sat down for dinner, I'd had a few more drinks and was fully saturated.

"Great V-neck sweater, cousin. Is that standard issue for all fraternity bros?" My older cousin, Jack, said playfully enough. He loved to lay into the East Coast, preppy, Dartmouth stereotype.

"Yeah, the frat sent it over, along with some beer pong balls and a toga. How about you? Still on summer break?"

It was a low blow. He'd never quite found his footing in college, struggling with grades and his own mental health issues, which would eventually be diagnosed. After a rocky first two years, he never returned for Fall Semester.

My mom leaned over to whisper in my ear, "Hey, David, what's going on? Have you maybe had too much to drink?"

"Oh, I dunno. Probably. But it's Christmas!"

"David, take it easy, now," my dad said, sharply, from two seats down.

"What am I doing wrong? This is what we do, right? Get a little drunk on Christmas? I thought that was the tradition."

"Cut the shit," he said.

"Why? You didn't!"

Another low blow. I knew he wouldn't be able to respond. I was untouchable in the space carved out for me by his old transgressions.

His lips tightened, his glare narrowed in. I'd seen that face a thousand times as a kid. It usually signaled that it was time for me to high tail it to my room. But I was no longer a child trapped in his house. I didn't have to run and hide. And so, I just smiled back.

But after that last taunt, the hollow satisfaction I felt gave way to guilt. I'd humiliated my cousin, made my parents seethe, and embarrassed my sisters. The rest of the table looked, at best, disappointed. It seemed that I'd taken up the tradition of ruining holiday dinners.

Chapter 2 - Come Out and Play

A couple months of dark winter passed. After that Christmas, I became more detached from my family than ever. They likely didn't recognize me anymore, though perhaps they recognized the addiction. I didn't call often, and I visited even less. Hearing them, seeing them—it made me feel shame for who I knew I was becoming. Dad, or something worse.

I grew thirstier. I wanted to drink more. More shots, more beers, more everything, more often. I started nights anxious and irritable, only relaxing after I drank enough to lose count. Fewer and fewer people could or would keep up with me. It had only been a few months since I last saw Will in Chicago. But because he was among the only drinking partners who kept pace with me, it felt much longer. Finally, the time for our quarterly tryst came around. This time, Will would head to California.

On the way to the airport, I brimmed once again, my body tingling at the perch atop the roller coaster.

"Will! My sweet prince!"

"Dave! Yeah, baby!"

He sounded excited, too. But when he got in the car, he had a look in his eyes that I didn't quite recognize. Something like apprehension or wariness. I hoped it was nothing—just my own insecurity about how much I expected him to drink with me. I needed him to be my counterpart more than ever. But the air between us in the car felt a few degrees different.

We headed back to the apartment while I chirped out details of the weekend I envisioned for us, including tickets to the Warriors that night. He smiled and moved fluidly enough through conversation about alcohol, basketball, and Scrabble. But I couldn't ward off the sense that something was amiss.

Annie gave us a lift to the Warriors game a few hours later. Halfway there, Will asked me from the back seat, "Did you remember the tickets?"

I turned around and stared at him sternly for a moment, feigning incredulity. But after I checked my pockets, I broke out in laughter. "As a matter of fact, I didn't."

Annie rolled her eyes. "Wow, you're off to a great start, guys!" She turned the car around at the next exit, and we headed back to our apartment. "I'm not giving you guys a ride all the way there this time. I'll take you to the subway and that's it, you dummies."

Annie double-parked while I sprinted inside to grab the abandoned tickets. I wasn't surprised I forgot them. I'd drunk a lot of Seagram's Black whiskey during the quick stop at our apartment after the airport.

Even though we'd paid a chunk for the tickets, I wasn't particularly distressed about missing part of the game. We were seeing Gilbert Arenas and the Wizards - not Kobe and the Lakers.

We had put the remainder of the whiskey into two flasks that Will brought with him. One with the Warriors' logo and one with the Celtics', his favorite team. They were made of cut-rate stainless steel with plastic team logos slapped on with glue.

"You know, these looked a lot better online." He'd said what I already thought.

"Hey, man, 'it's the thought', as they say. I love it."

Annie only took us as far as the subway, just as she'd warned. We'd missed half of the game already, but I didn't mind. Will and I were together, and we would drink all weekend. I didn't care what else we did or where.

"Bye, sweetie," I said to Annie before hopping out onto the sidewalk. "Thanks so much for the rides—both of them!"

"Have fun, boys. Please be safe. Seriously."

"We will, don't worry!" I promised as we trotted off down the subway steps.

We got through the ticketing station in record time because everyone already had their seats. We had the two flasks and had missed most of the game, but I told Will we should grab a couple of beers before we sat down. He was already hammered, but I still had a little way to go.

"We're fine," he said, with some noticeable weight behind it. "We've got the whiskey, and it's early. We're going to end up going out after this, too."

"Let's just get them so we have them, in case you want it later. We won't have to get up and miss any more of the game," I persisted. *And why the fuck are we even arguing about getting more alcohol?*

We normally went just about drink for drink. But tonight, he got wasted way ahead of schedule. I wondered if he hadn't been drinking as much since I'd last seen him and he'd lost some tolerance. Or perhaps he got drunk so easily because he'd been drinking *too* much?

Guilt hit me as soon as I realized that part of me might have preferred that. The line between companionship and complicity could be imprecise to me, at least when it came to my habit. In that moment, the selfish addict in me wanted Will to drink just to appease me, even if it was despite himself. That's the grip alcohol had over me—my best friend's well-being had to contend with my need for a hard-charging drinking partner.

We had almost made it to our seats when Will stumbled on the last couple of steps, nearly falling into someone's lap before I caught him. *Come on, man, lock it up.* I sank inside myself for the rest of the game, aggravated by the narrow but perceptible gap I felt between us. I drank more, faster, as I often did to stifle a troubling thought.

I drank the flask of whiskey and both pints of beer. By the fourth quarter, I'd gotten about as drunk as Will—nearly blacked out. We'd eventually arrived at the same place. *I'll turn this night around. It'll be just like always.*

III

How did we just lose to the Wizards? Jesus, Will is moving so damn slow. He doesn't have his glasses. Helpless without them. He looks like a kid lost at the fair. Get it together, man.

"Will! Shit! We forgot our new flasks!"

"They were like—ten bucks. I'll get you a new one. Promise."

"What if there's no others like it?"

"I think the factory might have cranked out more than one."

"Ha! There's my guy. Hey, come on, let's catch this next train."

"We're fine—what's the hurry?"

"I just don't want us to get stuck in line at the subway, that's all."

Because I don't want to let too much fucking time pass before we get the next drink—why do you think? He wouldn't have asked that a couple years ago. It shouldn't bother me. Shouldn't be a thing. But it is. What the fuck is going on with him? Why does he not want to get fucked up? He hasn't said anything about cutting back. He still drinks with me when we're on Skype. Or am I just too drunk to notice he's been slowing down? Maybe.

Where is he? Wow, he really is moving slow. There—his head. He's on the escalator. In a crowd. Oh, no—he just fell down. Hard. A couple people helping.

"I'll take him. Thanks so much for rescuing my friend!"

"You sure you guys are okay? That cut looks pretty bad, man."

Okay, Good Samaritan, mind your own fucking business. "Ay, ay, a scratch, a scratch!" *No laughs? Great reference, too bad.*

Shit. A lot of blood. Okay, I'm not pissed at you anymore, poor guy. He loves this jacket. Celtics colors. But there's nothing else to wrap his hand with. Not using my Monta Ellis jersey.

An older woman sitting across from us staring. Concerned, uncomfortable, both.

"Do you need some help? I think I might have some Band-Aids in my purse."

"It's worth a shot. Thank you."

"Take care of him. That doesn't look too good."

"We'll be fine, don't worry." *Everyone is getting on my fucking nerves.*

These things are tiny. I'm trying to do a good job. But I'm fucking hammered. And the train—the motherfucker won't stop shaking. What a mess. Criss-crossed little strips, already mostly soaked through. And not clean. At all. He's passed out. He can sleep until we get downtown. We're still going out tonight. Fuck his hand, he shouldn't have fallen.

"Will! We're here, come on."

Not moving. I'm gonna shake his damn head until he gets up.

"Dave," *Finally, fuck.* "Can you not shake my head anymore?" *Good, his eyelids fighting their way open. A smile.*

"I tried other stuff first, I swear! Okay, we're headed up another escalator. Don't fall, Sweet Prince."

Long valley of tall buildings and bright lights. There's energy out here tonight. A little buzz. I can feel it. I don't care where we go. The first bar that seems good. I just want some noise and commotion and drunk, rowdy people. This one will do.

A shot of Jägermeister and Red Bull for each of us. Maybe it will wake him up a bit.

"Who won the game?"

She must've seen my Monta Ellis jersey.

"Wizards – Unbelievable! Are you a Warriors fan?"

"Of course! Monta is my favorite player."

"Well, he kind of shit the bed tonight."

"You and your friend want a drink?" *Not flirting. Just want to drink. With whoever. Will is too far gone to keep up with me.*

"What do you think you're doing, bro?" *Her boyfriend, I guess. Tight black t-shirt, tighter black jeans, gold chain. Gross.*

"I said, why the fuck you talking to my girl, bro?"

Yes. Fun.

"She talked to me, *bro*." *Back to his girlfriend, like he's not even there.* "Anyways, as I was saying before this guy with the necklace here interrupted me, Monta was trash tonight, but—"

He's got the collar of my shirt. Clenching his fist. I've got his too, now. I can't hear what he's saying. Just smiling back. Blow his girlfriend a kiss, that'll make him nuts.

He's trying to land a punch. Not gonna happen. I'm taller. My arm is still outstretched with his collar clenched in my hand. His swings are falling far short. Keep smiling.

Bouncers pulling us apart. They yank me all the way outside. Don't resist, it's fine. I had my fun. Will doesn't even realize what's happening. Why'd they let the other guy stay and not me? We were both acting like assholes. Probably because he's got girls with him and I've got the guy with Band-Aids all over his hand.

Will is coherent again. That episode woke him up a bit.

"Dave—are we okay?"

"Ha, yes. Don't worry." *I have my arm around his shoulders, and he has one on mine. It feels good. The irritation I felt towards him, it's gone. I was being too sensitive and—shit, what's this?*

A different hand on my other shoulder. Digging into me, pulling, and whirling me around. This is a big person, with a big, fat paw. Cops. And they're fucking huge. They're stepping right into me, pressing their fingers into my chest.

"Give me some identification!"

"What did we do—what the fuck is going on?" *Did someone at the bar call the police? Will looks scared.*

I'm sorry, Will.

"Shut the fuck up and empty your pockets!"

They're pushing me. Backpedaling into a parked car. Nowhere to go.

"Now!"

Wallets. Whatever else we got. But they're still pushing us with their fat fucking hands. You motherfuckers. I know what you're doing. Don't fight back. They want a reason to arrest me. But I'm losing control. They've got me by the collar, yanking me around. That animal in me... I'm losing it.

"Don't fucking touch us!"

My wrists. My head slams into the top of a car. That hurt.

"Get the fuck off of us! We didn't do shit!"

Trying to get out of this hold they've got me in. Thrashing. People watching. I didn't want this. But now I do. I can't turn back. Letting this animal out of me feels good. Pushing. Pulling. But they're too strong. I'm pinned against the car again.

Shit. Cuffs.

Back of their big van. Cuffing me to a seat in the back. Still kicking, cursing, thrashing. I'll kick the metal bars on this window until they fucking break. One of these fuckers is smirking at me.

"Fuck you!" *Fucking asshole cop.*

Been in this van for at least an hour. There's a few of us so far. New friends for the night. Some of them look scared. Some don't. Not their first time. I don't feel it yet, but I know something is coming after this anger and this alcohol wear off. Guilt. It's gonna set in fucking hard. I'm dreading it. I'll have to explain this to Annie. I've never been arrested before. What am I even going to say? That it wasn't our fault? That the cops picked on us? Sure. But she won't buy any of it. My bosses at work won't know, I don't think, unless they keep me here for more than one night. Shit. Will they? I hadn't thought of that. This is getting out of control. Dig this hole deeper.

The animal, it wants me to self-destruct.

"Fuck you, assholes!" *Kicking these metal bars on the windows some more.*

The station. A big, gray cement facility. Taking everyone off the van. Except me. They didn't say too much to me while I acted up. But now I'll pay for it. An example. Great. Fuck you, pigs.

Two big officers. One has my ankles. The other has my head. I'm getting dragged down the aisle like a log. Thrown onto the pavement. Picking me back up, propping me up on my feet. Wrists trapped behind me. Their hands on the back of my head. Shit, here it comes. The cement wall is hurtling towards me. Payback is a—

My head is hanging. How long was I out? Feet flopping across the dirty floor. Getting dragged like a knocked-out boxer. Where the hell is my other shoe?

It's ugly in here. The lights are harsh. Piercing. It smells like the streets. The walls are yellow but used to be white. The floor is sticky and stained with... everything.

The two officers are passing us off to the staff and an on-site nurse. She's firing off intake questions to everyone, one at a time. The two cops that dragged me off the bus are hovering around me.

"How's your head feeling, boy? You fucked with the wrong shift tonight!"

That one's badge says Marquez.

"If you're not careful, we're gonna throw you upstairs with the inmates. The big boys up there are going to split you open."

This one's Johnson.

"You'd like that, I bet, assholes."

But they're just laughing at me some more. It's my turn for the nurse.

"Are you injured?"

"Yeah. Look at my head. These two smashed my head into a fucking wall."

"No, he had that cut when we picked him up." *Johnson is laughing while he says it.*

"Sounds like you had that when they picked you up. Where is your shoe?" *She's smirking. You're in on the joke, too? Great.*

"Probably in the parking lot they dragged me through."

"No, he only had one shoe when we picked him up."

"Sounds like you only had one shoe when they picked you up." *She's grinning.*

"One more question. Do you take any medication?"

"Yes. Psychiatric medication. And I need it in the morning."

"Okay, so you take some psychological drugs, got it."

Idiot. "There's no such thing as psychological drugs. Aren't you a nurse?"

"Got it. Psychological drugs."

More laughter, the kind from bullies that have a weaker kid backed into a corner. I've really fucked up. The alcohol's burning off. I don't like what I am. My hands—they look different. Far away, like they're someone else's.

They throw me into a different cell than Will. I haven't seen him since his intake, which he sleep-walked through. I hope no one is bothering him. He just wanted to go home. You're stuck in this now because of me. I'm so sorry, Will.

It's almost three in the morning. Most of the other guys in here have passed out. A few, like me, are pacing around. It'll be too hard to sleep. My heart rate is all jacked up. The dent on my head hurts like hell. I'm too fucking mad at these cops. Johnson and Marquez. SFPD's finest motherfuckers.

But who am I kidding? It was me. All me. And, in a few more hours, I know I'll be flooded with guilt, embarrassment, and dread of having to tell Annie.

An hour or two of sleep would be nice. But I don't think I'm gonna get it.

Chapter 4 - A Permanent Stain

The big metal gate to the cell swung open at about eight in the morning. Groups of five or six at a time got released every half an hour or so. I didn't get called with the first group. Or the second. Not with the third or fourth group, either. I was alone. I knew what they were doing—bleeding it out. Johnson and Marquez had long gone, sleeping cozily somewhere. But they'd left a parting gift for me, of course. They had the staff on the morning shift keep me locked up. I knew they could hold me up to twenty-four hours without charging me. I just hoped they wouldn't. I grew nervous that they might keep me for the weekend. Another hour. Noon. I started getting desperate. I didn't have any adrenaline—or alcohol—left in me. I was just sad and crushed into submission.

A few hours later, another shift changed. I hoped the new crew wasn't *also* in on the joke. When a new guard passed by the cell, I told her I had some daily medications that I really had to take. It was true, of course. But using my medicine to get myself out of jail? I wasn't proud of it. I was, however, out of options.

"Hang on a minute. Let me see what's going on with you," she said before disappearing down the hall.

I figured she went to check those immaculate medical records the intake nurse had logged the night before, to see if I was lying about the medications.

"All right, we're letting you out of here."

"Thanks, I appreciate it."

"Don't fuck around with those cops. That was stupid. You're lucky we didn't hit you with resisting arrest. It's probably only because they didn't want to stick around doing more paperwork."

"You're right. Thanks. And there won't be a next time."

I kept my head down as the staff checked me out. I feared some other guard would run over and tell her to keep my ass in there until Johnson and Marquez got back that night. She handed me off to a staff member who gave me a yellow paper bag. The contents: one phone, one wallet, one belt, and one shoe.

I got out to the street to find it gray and drizzling. I was glad for it. I didn't want the sun shining into my bloodshot eyes. And I didn't want to see people looking the way they do on a nice, sunny Saturday. With the smidge of battery left in my phone, I called a cab. I felt far too ashamed to call Annie. No, I texted her, like a coward, to tell her that I was sorry I fucked up and was out of jail and headed home.

I didn't know how much of this she would put up with. I was two-timing her. But not with another girl—I was having an affair with booze. I'd rationalized that I could do both if I could just get my relationship with alcohol under control. But I couldn't think about it right then. I stamped out the thought as fast as I could before the spark of anxiety turned into a fire.

When I finally trudged in, she looked at me. "Will is fine. He's asleep in the bedroom. I'm not staying. I just wanted to see you in one piece. Now, I'm getting out of here for a while."

Those were the only words she had for me. The rest, she told me silently. She had beautiful eyes, but I was making them sad and tired.

"I'm sorry, babe. I don't even know what to say."

"Good, because I don't want to hear anything right now."

"I understand. I am really, really sorry."

I collapsed on the couch and closed my eyes, but I couldn't sleep. I felt completely fatigued, yet my mind raced. I was trapped in an uncomfortable crevice between panic and exhaustion. I could feel the restlessness crawling on my skin. Needing distraction, I started flipping through my phone, wondering if I'd taken any pictures. Not many—I had been too drunk to remember to snap more than a few. I found two or three that Annie took of me and Will with our arms around each other before we left for the game. Then a couple of us with our crappy Celtics and Warriors flasks. Not much after that. I noticed one more, though.

At first, I couldn't tell what it was. I zoomed in and out on it, then flipped it from portrait to landscape, trying to decipher the dark and blurry image. I thought maybe I just tapped the button by accident. But then I made the picture out, and I felt a nauseating sting. Right then, Will stumbled into the living room, rubbing his eyes.

"Hey, man. Are you okay?" I asked. "I'm so sorry. I didn't mean for any of that to happen."

"Yeah, I know you didn't."

"We should have just gone home after the game. I don't know why I couldn't see that—I was just out of my head."

"Those cops—they could have really fucked you up. Or have you still in jail and charging you. You can't do that shit, Dave. You're lucky to even be here right now."

I nodded in acknowledgement. But I didn't have any words. *Will, I'm scared, but I don't know what to do.*

"I love you, bro. I just don't want you to get hurt. Are you taking your meds?"

"Yeah, I usually do," I said, "most of the time."

"Do you think that's what's making you get so aggressive when you drink? The pills? You didn't used to get so mad. I've never seen you like that. When we used to get drunk, you would usually just get—I don't know. It was just different. Easy and fun, and we'd fuck around and eventually pass out. And then, you know, sometimes you'd piss your pants." He usually knew the right time to say something funny.

His joke forced a laugh out of me, releasing the tension building in my face, shoulders, and clenched fists. "Honestly, I really don't know. Maybe it's the meds. We're definitely not supposed to mix alcohol with them. But fuck, man, maybe it's just something in me."

"What do you mean?"

It was scary to tread this terrain. "I mean, like, when I get like that, it almost feels like I'm not even myself, like there's some fucking animal taking over. Once those cops put their hands on me, I wasn't even thinking anymore. It was a different person."

It was taking him some time to respond, so I kept going, needing to confide in my best friend. "These days, after I've been drinking a lot, sooner or later I just get angry. Anything sets it off. Someone looking at me the wrong way. I almost *want* someone to look at me the wrong way. I want to fight. I want to get hurt. Make a mess. Make chaos. I don't know, man, I didn't use to be like that. Just would drink, laugh, and, like you said, probably piss myself."

"I hear you, man. Well, what are you going to do about it? Maybe it's something you can work on and figure out? I think you should at least start by talking to your doctor about it. Don't you think?"

"Yeah, I know. I need to. I will. I don't like the guy, but I'll talk to him," I conceded, before redirecting the conversation. "Oh, by the way, take a look at this," I said, thrusting my cell phone in his face. "It turns out we took some pictures last night."

"Uh oh," he said, knowing I needed to change the subject. "This should be good." He stared at the grainy, blurry image for a few long seconds. Suddenly his eyes widened, and his mouth opened. "Jesus, Dave," he said.

"I know, man. Not good. Not good at all."

When we arrived late to the game last night, there were two Oakland Police Department motorcycles parked outside the arena with the police helmets on the handlebars. In the stupidest of impulses, I'd hopped on a police officer's bike, put on their helmet, and pretended to ride, swiveling the bars left and right. There was even a baton in its holster that I took out and wielded around in the air. I had shoved my phone into Will's hand and made him take a picture.

"I don't look bad in that helmet. Maybe I could be a cop if the real estate thing doesn't pan out?"

I attempted the joke to evade embarrassment and fear. I knew it wasn't funny, but I didn't know what else to do. If I admitted my problem was serious, I'd have to do something about it. So, instead, I joked. We laughed awkwardly. I laughed to lie to myself. He laughed to catch my fall.

Our trip to the airport on Sunday was quiet. I was preoccupied in the driver's seat, nervous that our relationship would imminently change after this fucked-up trip. I feared he wouldn't want to drink with me anymore, or, at least, not with the total abandon we were used to. I feared he might want to distance himself from me, as to not risk being collateral damage to my self-destruction. I feared things would now be different.

"Pretty crazy weekend," I offered. "I'm sorry again, bro. That was way over the top."

"It certainly was unexpected, that's for sure. But hey, man—just try to learn from it and make sure something like that never happens again."

"I know. Definitely. Thanks."

We got into the departures drop off and both hopped out.

"Okay. Get some rest on the flight. Love you, Sweet Prince."

"Love you too. I'll let you know when I land."

After a hug, I hung back and watched him head through the automatic doors. He had his duffel bag slung on one shoulder and, on the other, his favorite jacket. I could see where the blood from his fall on the escalator marred the Celtics green. He thought it might come out with a Tide pen and a good scrub. But I knew the stain wasn't going anywhere.

Part Seven

Chapter 1 - La Farmacia

After I left Will at the airport, I remembered Annie and I had plans to go to a dinner party at a friend's house. Feeling that I had just betrayed my best friend, I wanted to pivot and find approval from others. On top of that, I was avoiding being confronted by Annie. I called her from the car to see if she still wanted to go. I didn't even know if she would answer, much less want to do anything together.

"Babe, are you there?" I asked. She'd picked up but said nothing.

"Yeah?"

"Did you still want to go to Lara's for her dinner thing? I think we said we were gonna go. If you want, I can just come home, and we can talk."

After another pause, "No, let's go. I'll meet you there."

"I can pick you up. I just dropped off Will."

"I'll meet you there."

I made a stop at the store, knowing I couldn't show up empty-handed. Without thinking much about it, I picked up what I usually brought to a party. But when I got there with a case of thirty Bud Lights, it looked painfully out of place. Hardly anyone was drinking. Just a few glasses of red wine and some craft beers. It was Sunday, after all. I felt the sharp embarrassment of missing something that was obvious to everyone else.

I saw it out of the corner of my eye, two of our friends looking at each other a certain way. It was a subtle cue, but it pierced me like the sharpest insult. Right then, I knew they'd talked about this before. Me drinking too much, at the wrong time, or in the wrong places. Or, more likely, all of the above.

I felt anger at them for that fucking look. I felt loathing toward myself for embarrassing Annie. And I felt fear. Fear that I was on an island that was being evacuated. Every time I looked up, the land was shrinking around me. Fewer people wanted to hang out with me. Annie was growing wary of me. *What if eventually I'm the only one left?*

Then, for a moment, the animal in me perked up, pushing the fear and self-loathing out and leaving only the anger. *They're wrong. I'm fine. They're just boring, and I like to have fun. What is wrong with that? I don't care if I see them again. I don't care if I see anyone that judges me or gives that fucking look! I'm not going to leave drinking behind, so I'll leave them behind instead.* But the defiance passed. That wasn't what I wanted. I didn't want to push away these friends, Will, or, most of all, Annie in favor of a reckless drinking habit.

I felt an impetus to change after that weekend. I'd just spent the night in jail, only to show up to a dinner party with a case of beers, for fuck's sake. I'd put Will in jail, embarrassed myself in front of friends, and put a tenuous, uncomfortable distance between Annie and me. That embarrassment, and the fear of screwing up my relationship, served to corral me for a while. I became more aware of every sip people saw me take. I felt like their eyes always trained on me, a precursor to their quiet, but no less thorny, judgments. So, for a couple months, I didn't drink as hard. I still had whiskey or beer most nights, but just enough to get my fix. Not enough to trigger angry, wild outbursts.

I settled into a groove of drinking often but managing to not humiliate myself or get into trouble. I started to feel like I'd hit the mark. A balancing act I thought might give me what I wanted—alcohol, without the alienation.

Annie began to feel better around me. Safer. She grew optimistic that the night of the Warriors game was an isolated occurrence—just a bad mistake that I wouldn't let happen again. Her eyes, when they looked at me, changed back from despondent to bright and green. She let her guard down. When my five-year reunion at Dartmouth arrived, she didn't worry too much. I'd modeled pretty good behavior. Besides, with everyone else getting blasted, and the school sanctioning a certain amount of bedlam, I couldn't possibly manage too much undue mischief.

I felt giddy. I'd been looking forward to it for over a year. I couldn't wait to melt into two full days spent only with the hardest drinking buddies, whom I hadn't seen in a few years. I could cast the dinner party crowd—the ones that scoffed at my thirty-pack of Bud Light—aside for a few days. I'd been behaving better and deserved to briefly shed restraint, I told myself.

Annie and I went out to dinner the night before I left. I tried to focus on her. I tried to focus on her face and lips and eyes as she talked, and on the words coming out of her mouth. But I could only think of the upcoming bender. We were sharing a table, only feet apart. But I simply wasn't there.

Over the course of dinner, I thought about whether she could see what was really behind my eyes. Maybe she could sense that she was sharing me with my consuming desire to escape into a fucking sea of booze. For an overwhelming moment, before I drowned it in a big gulp of wine, I wondered how long she would let me split my love between her and my habit.

Back home after dinner, as I tossed ratty clothes into a bag, Annie caught me packing my old digital Canon 3.2-megapixel point-and-shoot. Same one I'd had since before phones had cameras built in. I was the last person our age still hanging on to one of the old relics. I'd made a point to avoid embracing the growing conformity of iPhone integration.

"Why are you bringing that? You do know it's not even gonna make it back, right?"

"Come on, I can make it through a weekend without losing my stuff!"

"I think it's a good thing you're taking it. If you lose it, it's for the best."

"Hey, they take better pictures than these phones do."

"No," she quickly hit back. "They take better pictures than *your* phone does."

I looked down at my first-generation iPhone, then back up at her. I fogged the cracked screen with my breath, and then treated it to a little shining with my sleeve. We laughed together and shared a moment of ease. She didn't seem overly nervous about my trip, perhaps confident enough I could make it through the weekend without incident. What could possibly go wrong?

Adrenaline whipped through me as James and I got out of the airport in Boston. We had flown out one day early so we could spend a night with Taylor, Noah, and a few of our other college friends who lived Back East. My body knew, as much as my brain did, that it was only a cab ride away from getting fully saturated in alcohol. I was like a dog that knew he was about to get a treat—bouncy, giddy, salivating.

The rain poured when we got to Taylor's Boston apartment. He answered the door looking like he always did, with boat shoes and a Brooks Brother polo tucked into plaid shorts.

"Are you going golfing or sailing?" I asked.

"Dave! How are you, brother?" Taylor beamed a huge grin and put his arms out for a hug. He poured James and me each a Maker's Mark on the rocks. *Classy.*

Taylor's apartment was nicer than any I knew. He worked in venture capital, which apparently afforded him a brownstone flat right on the Boston Commons. He even had one of the prized, reserved parking spots underneath the park, which I'd heard cost about five hundred bucks a month. That was more than the lease on my Mazda and a month's worth of gas.

The flat, the job, the BMW, and even the parking spot, all inspired a bit of good-natured envy. But what I envied about Taylor more than the stuff he had was that he had both success and still partied a ton. As far as I could tell, he'd managed to be kicking ass at work and still did plenty of drugs and alcohol. *I should move here and start hanging out with Taylor. Maybe he can give me a job in venture capital, whatever the hell that is.*

After a couple hours of hasty drinking and updates on work, girlfriends, and sports, we were good and drunk. James took out some Vicodin he'd gotten on a recent trip to Mexico. We waited before expressing skepticism of the quality of the pills and, sure enough, the blissful tranquility of hard alcohol and painkillers soon washed over us.

My mind rarely got so quiet or peaceful as that evening. Even when I was off booze for a few days and took my meds right on time every morning, the animal still disparaged me. *Do better—at everything. No, pick a fight—with everyone. Forget it—you're a fuck-up—just keep drinking.* But that night, with my old friends around me and a flood of alcohol and opioids zipping through my brain, the animal stayed dormant in its dark cave.

I lay down and slept in the silent eye of my storm.

Chapter 2 - Don't Turn Off the Lights

We all piled into Taylor's BMW around lunchtime and headed north, our shoulders smashed up against one another's. We looked like gangly, young boys getting shuttled to soccer practice. By the time we got to New Hampshire, the rain and clouds had cleared and revealed a beautiful summer day. The granite cliffs towered over us and every tree bloomed full of color. The Connecticut River—my home every Fall and Spring afternoon—flowed with glistening, clean water.

The campus looked exquisite as we pulled up to the green quad. Every building, landmark, or artifact prompted a memory. The green and white Dartmouth Hall reminded me of my favorite class, American poetry, where we read Whitman, Thoreau, and Frost. The red brick dean's building reminded me of sitting in front of the housing dean's office until we got Alex's room reassigned, after he'd walked in the night before to find his roommate masturbating on *his* bed. The huge athletic center reminded me of the extra workouts Will and I did to sweat out surplus alcohol and angst before team practice.

Before getting to our fraternity, we stopped at Stinson's Market. Five years later, the little corner store still thrived. It was called a "market," but they sold mainly beer, cups, and everything else needed for beer pong and parties. If they sold food, nobody ever noticed. The store itself was tiny, but the loading area and cold storage in the back were huge—the perfect layout for a sizable distribution business. Stinson's had kept Dartmouth kids wasted for decades.

With as many thirty-packs as we could carry, we descended back into our fraternity basement for the first time in five years. My skin tingled. This would be our sanctuary for the next few days. It looked the same, smelled the same, felt the same. The Greek letters we painted were still intact, except for some intermittent touch up work that had been done. Everything looked just as we left it. Perfect. Frozen in time. We saw the school's motto, *Vox Clamantis en Deserto*, still scrawled on the wall. *A Voice Cries Out in the Wilderness.*

A couple of hours evaporated quickly as we made our way through a case or two of Keystone Light. We had to go to the reunion dinner, one of the few official events I planned to attend. I saw no reason to stop drinking. Shit, at least the registration fee included an open bar.

But my friends slowed down some, which annoyed me. They were socializing more, drinking less. The high I had felt mere moments before melted away and left me embarrassed. I felt different, like an other. Like everybody else had turned left where I'd turned right. They were moving forward and upward into graduate degrees, money, and professional reputation. I hadn't chased these things—just the next drink.

I felt my mind racing when I spoke with people I used to know. All their innocuous questions stung me like little pinpricks. What I did for work. Whether I had thought of graduate school. *There are miles between us. You can't imagine what my life has been since you last saw me. And I can't imagine yours. Fuck this conversation—I'm not here for this. I need another drink.*

Finally, dinner wrapped up, and we retreated back to the basement. Bothered that many of my friends were less drunk than I wanted them to be, I continued to shove drink after drink in their mitts. We turned the stereo on loud, putting in a playlist we made on the car ride up. It blared the same songs we used to listen to—terrible boy bands, Journey, and Noah's favorite, "Don't Turn off the Lights," by Enrique Iglesias. We sang, played, and drank. I had as much alcohol as I could hold down, with no one saying I'd had too many. It felt like freedom, not the prison of dependence and self-medication it actually was.

Over the next couple of hours, the party grew. More old faces. Some I'd been close with. Others I wasn't. But it didn't matter. We were all there, sharing a moment. One that was ephemeral, though not trivial. A moment from another time, years before, borrowed and shared again. I felt free from the anxiety consuming me, free from the voice in my head that always struck me down.

I felt happiness—and I believed it was real.

James, Noah, and the guys were still asleep when I woke up. I had plenty of time before the planned crew team alumni row at nine. I stopped for a coffee at Lou's Cafe, which I remembered being much, much better.

I wasn't in great shape at that time. The same appeared true of my old teammates, though likely for different reasons. Some toiled in med school libraries. Others worked eighty hours climbing the ranks. Not me. I just drank a lot and took anti-depressants.

I felt a sting of embarrassment when I arrived last. I thought nine a.m. meant nine a.m.

"Boys!" I shouted as I blasted open the green double doors to the boathouse. "Let's do this!"

Someone shouted, "Hey, Dave! We were worried you wouldn't make it!"

I knew the comment wasn't meant to jab me in the stomach, but it did. "Wouldn't miss it, man. I miss *you*, though."

I looked out at the water—flat and smooth. Perfect conditions, just like the first time we beat Brown. We locked our oars into the gunnels and strapped our feet in.

Kate, our old coxswain, hadn't lost her touch. "Okay, you fat motherfuckers. Just because you're all out of shape now, don't think I'm taking it easy on you!"

We summoned the synchrony we'd perfected five years prior and coupled it with whatever residual stamina still lingered in our legs. It was a surprisingly refreshing result. The boat clicked along with a retired, but still familiar, rhythm.

On the good practices, when the river was smooth and we rowed well, it was so quiet we could hear our blades cut in and out of the water on every stroke. The silence in between indicated near-perfect technique, rhythm, and balance. Five years removed, we still managed to find that silence—at least until everyone's breathless gasps drowned it out.

Our boat was balanced and steady enough that I could close my eyes and sink into each long squeeze of the legs and heave of the back and arms. I remembered that, for me, the only thing more prevalent than the searing pain of rowing was the peace. Out on the water, I didn't hear a voice. I didn't need a drink. I wished we could stay out there until sundown.

We planned to take four laps on our old course at three-quarters effort. A challenging but manageable workout. By the time we got to the third, though, complaints came from all directions.

"Okay, this is fun and all, but I'm going to throw up if we don't stop soon," someone said. "I haven't worked out since… fuck, I don't even know."

A small chorus of agreement followed. *No, not just yet.* I almost said it out loud before catching myself. They didn't know that this was the best I had felt in years. They didn't know how much I needed it. I couldn't let them know, of course. It wasn't their problem. They were only out on the water for a small taste of old memories.

The big class dinner on the second night was almost formal, much nicer than I cared for. I wanted to bail but couldn't convince anyone to go with me. It was the big event of the weekend, after all. There were a couple of speeches by whoever was our class president and probably whoever was in charge of alumni fundraising.

I drank as much free wine and beer as I could while the speeches and slideshows unfolded, quickly hurling myself towards another blackout. After dinner, we went back to the basement of our fraternity. A few of the guys decided not to come and just turn in early on our last night. This made me seethe. But at least it was only the rowdiest of us who remained. I'd be accompanied by the people that really wanted to get blitzed.

Who knows who started it, or why. Maybe me. *Probably* me. But after a few beer-pong games, a few of us started wrestling and throwing light punches. We laughed as we threw each other into the big plywood tables, shouted as we hurled rubber trash cans back and forth. We howled as we drunkenly landed soft punches onto one another's anesthetized chins.

Everyone relented after the five-minute bout. Not me, though—or, rather, not the animal crawling out of its cave. It wanted a turn, too. I kept pushing Chris, less playfully, more forcefully, and with a sneering grin on my face. Chris was big and strong and we all remembered his legendary fights out on the Dartmouth hockey rink. I knew I could provoke him.

He resisted, at first. But when I tagged him with a sharp jab across the cheek, he quickly put me down. I got up and leapt at him, but he dropped me again. I reveled in it with a sick, masochistic glee. Once more, I dove at him, throwing a couple punches to his body before he slammed me a third time. He meant it to be the last time. He wasn't amused anymore. He walked outside, perhaps thinking I was done.

But I flew at him again in the parking lot, lowering my shoulder into his chest. He planted his feet and let me dig into him. Then, he quickly wrapped my head up with a strong, right arm. I tried to break free, hurling my knees and hands at him. He spun me around, positioning himself behind me, and cinched his arm even tighter around my neck, until I couldn't breathe. That should have been my cue to submit and put a stop to the beating I was taking. But I kept flailing at him, now with heels and elbows. *I've never been choked unconscious. I want to see what it's like.*

"Come on man, just stop fighting!" Someone shouted at me. "This isn't funny anymore, Dave. You're getting yourself hurt."

His arm tightened around my throat every time I shot my elbow backwards into his ribs. He had my head cocked back, toward the sky. I suddenly noticed the vivid white stars up above me. *Out here in New Hampshire, away from the city, they're so much brighter.*

Then, slowly, from the periphery inwards, darkness drowned them out. The sound faded, too. I heard silence as the last few remaining stars were blotted out. My hands stopped prying at his arm and finally fell to my sides. *This feels good. It's peaceful and soft.*

And then the lights turned off.

III

Was I just asleep? They're all shouting at me.

"Dave! Dave!"

"Did Chris tap out?"

"What the fuck is wrong with you, man? Are you okay?" *Chris is laughing. Helping me up. A big bear hug.*

Big squeeze, I feel closer to him. "I feel fucking great."

Chris keeps looking at me. Inspecting me. "You're crazy, man. Let's go back down—oh, fuck."

Shit. Police. Everybody is scattering and heading to their rooms, ready to call it quits for the night. No, fuck no. The cops can't just come in here and rip my night away from me. This is ours, don't fucking touch it.

"Come on over here. Let's just sort this out and get you boys on your way home."

I tie my ripped shirt around my head. "Chase me, motherfuckers!"

Yes. They're running after me. Through the parking lot. Hurdle over these tables and lawn chairs. I'm faster. They must be long gone. But my legs aren't holding steady. Barely keeping my balance. Shit. Crashing to the ground. Laughing, I can't help it.

"What's so goddamn funny, asshole?" *Two of them stand me up and pin me, face first, against a brick wall of a dorm.*

"I think I used to live in this one."

One of the cops is older. Looks tired. But this other one. Young. Wiry. So eager. I can feel it in his grip. Almost shaking me. Shaved head. Pants tucked into fucking combat boots. "What are you trying to be, a Navy SEAL?"

His eyes are drilling into me. Lips are rigid. "Oh, you have jokes?"

My arm is cranked up behind me, towards my neck. He's leaning into it. Trying to make it hurt. Not laughing anymore. Motherfucker. A sting from his fingernails digging into my wrist. Sharp pain in my shoulder. I'm gonna fucking explode. My free hand, prying myself away from this wall.

"Let's fucking go, assholes! See what you can do."

"If you don't stay still, I'm going to empty this right into your fucking eyes!" *Shit. His pepper spray is an inch from my face.*

Maybe I should stop. I've been sprayed before. It sucked. He's got my wrist again. Pulling, whirls me around. Some kind of quick move. They've got me flattened on the ground. And there's a pointy knee in my back. Fuck. That was quick.

"Pepper spray? That was a pussy move, you fuckers." *Only a corner of my mouth is talking. The rest of it is eating dirt.*

"You're under arrest…"

Here come the metal handcuffs. I'm done. I don't care anymore. There's a silence. The chaos and anger in my head, they're fading away. It's time to let my body just go limp. I'm sinking into the ground. Maybe I can just fucking disappear into the earth. What the fuck is wrong with me? What did I just do, and why did I do it? I let the animal inside me take over. And now it's finished with me. Leaving me in a heap.

I'll stay quiet and compliant in the car. Panic is setting into my chest. What am I going to tell Annie? Can I keep it from her? My friends will know. Everyone here will know. Are they going to think that I'm fucking insane? That I've lost my mind and I'm just a junkie alcoholic? A lost cause?

Pulling me out, booking me, and putting me in a cell. There's no one else here. Of course, there fucking isn't. They let me use the phone to call someone. James. He picks up. God bless you for answering at six in the morning.

"Hey, man. It's Dave."

"Dude, what number are you calling me from?"

"Uh, jail, actually. Sorry."

"What the fuck—never mind. Just sit tight. Don't fuck around."

"Thanks, man. I won't. Sorry, James."

He shows up fast. Eyes are bloodshot and bleary. He gives the clerk some money. "At least bail in New Hampshire is only fifty bucks."

Thanks for breaking the ice, brother.

"I'll pay you back next time I see an ATM."

"Ha, yeah, you're damn right you will. So, what the hell happened, man?" *He's whispering.*

"I don't know. I just lost my head when those cops showed up. And then one of them got so aggressive, and I couldn't keep my cool." *Also, I have a fucking disease, I'm an addict, and I like feeling pain.*

Officer walking over with a yellow paper bag. Hands me my stuff. Finally, we can get the hell out of here.

"Hey, hold on, man—what the hell is going on, where's all my things?"

"This is all you had on you, man. Now get the fuck out of here."

"*Bullshit, man, no way!*" *No wallet or phone or keys. Just a tin of Skoal tobacco and a ping-pong ball. The cop is ignoring me. Probably telling the truth. No one here wants my empty wallet or my cracked iPhone 1.*

"You'll get a notice in the mail regarding your court date."

"Okay, okay. I fucking get it."

"If you don't report to court, we'll put out a warrant for arrest. Do you understand?"

"Sure. Just let me the fuck out of here."

Chapter 4 - We Need to Talk

I woke up from a couple hour nap somewhere over the mountain states after some terrible sleep. My body was exhausted from getting my ass kicked a couple different times, yet my brain was agitated and buzzed with static noise. That's what the guilt sounded like sometimes— scratchy, whiny static. James and I were on a flight back together, fortunately. I didn't want to be alone.

I was quickly realizing what had been hidden in plain fucking sight: I'd transformed. Everyone could see it. Even James and Chris and my other friends—guys that still drank a lot themselves— surely looked at me differently. I was the one that didn't stop drinking when everyone else did. The one that didn't recognize when it was the wrong time or place. The one that always took it way too fucking far.

Even at a five-year college reunion, an event basically designed for everyone to get fucked up, I'd still managed to separate myself in all the wrong ways. Some kids showed up to gleam and glow about the fellowships they'd earned or the startups they'd founded. Not me. I showed up to get my ass hauled to jail.

I wish we could have one more night. I'd show people that I can be fun without drinking. But I'm not sure if that's even true.

Ever since settling in San Francisco, mere months after getting out of Butler Hospital, I'd steadily tread deeper into my habit. One more drink each night. One more night each week. Addiction grows with a devious and surprising subtlety. And when my drinking accelerated, no one told me I let it get out of control. Why should they? It wasn't their job. But I mistook their silence as tacit approval.

Even Annie didn't tell me I drank too much until it was right in front of our faces. I couldn't blame her. I had gone to great lengths to conceal my heaviest, ugliest drinking. I used every little trick—nursing a secret flask in bathrooms, stopping at a neighboring bar before a dinner date, or simply just waiting her out, until she fell fast asleep. She surely had caught on to some of it, but not all.

She knew when I was drinking, but she didn't quite know how grotesque it could get. She hadn't seen me writhing, thrashing, and twisting through blackouts and ugly, angry benders. She didn't know just how much pain I tried to suppress. She couldn't see the dark, morbid images that plagued my mind when I was sober. The stuff I submerged in alcohol. Of course, she was probably the one person who could help me the most.

But I was ready. I wanted to talk, if she'd be willing to listen. I planned to tell her what happened over the weekend when she picked me up at the airport. But I needed to confess much more. I needed to let her know I was scared of who I was becoming—or who I'd already *become*—and wanted to find a way back before I lost her.

And at the thought of the impending conversation, the seats on the plane suddenly felt particularly tiny. My heart raced while my restless limbs felt trapped in place. Confining my space even more, James' big head had flopped onto my shoulder. His chin and tongue hung loosely, twitching with each snore. I wanted to shake him off. But I still owed him fifty bucks and a huge favor. He could park his noggin on my shoulder for the rest of the flight if he needed to.

After we crawled out of our tiny seats and dragged our tired bodies through the airport terminal, we stepped outside into the brisk San Francisco evening. I took a deep breath of the crisp air and felt something like relief when I exhaled. The anticipation of finally being honest with Annie felt good.

A few minutes after James stepped into a cab, Annie picked me up at the curb. When I saw her Jeep, a quick, nervous reflex told me I should have taken the subway home. *Are you really ready to have this conversation with her right now, man?* But I wasn't going to let myself chicken out. I knew I needed to start talking before it was too late. But as soon as I got into the car, I didn't have the chance to begin.

"What the heck happened?" Her tone was sharp.

What? But how do you know?

Then, as if she'd just read my mind, "Kelsey called me."

James' fucking girlfriend called you?

"I was going to tell you everything, just so you know. I was literally about to start this conversation."

"Sure."

"You don't believe me."

"I don't know, honestly. But you're going to tell me now. This is getting scary for me. Not to mention—fucking embarrassing, man."

"I just—I don't know, babe, I blacked out, and then I couldn't control anything. I got into a brawl, and it started as just having fun. But then some switch flipped. And I wasn't in control anymore. And then these cops showed up, and I—"

"I don't get it. Wasn't everyone else drunk? How were you the *one* person that—I don't understand."

"You're right. I don't know. It wasn't even me making the decisions, it was—I don't know—it feels like there's an animal that's buried inside me, and he comes out and takes over. I think some weird part of me wants to get hurt. Wants to take punishment. Chris choked me unconscious. It's so fucked up, but—I liked it. After that I should have just gone home, but I wanted more, so I made trouble with the cops until they kicked my ass. It's like I'm not the same person at all. I change."

"Yes," she said, softly. "That's what it looks like. To your friends. To me. But what are you going to do about it?"

"I don't know. But I know I don't want to keep going like this. I'm worried I'm going to fuck things up with us. I don't want you to leave me. I'm putting all this space between us, and I want to fix it, but—"

"But *what?*"

"I'm worried that the person you fell in love with, maybe he's gone."

"No. He's not gone. But you're right, I can't wait forever, either. It's too hard to watch from up close. I don't want to have to wonder where you are on the weekends. I can't be in a relationship where I'm scared you might have ended up in jail." After a pause, she added, "Or something worse."

Immediately, I imagined her getting a call that I'd killed myself driving drunk. I didn't always care what happened to me. But when she said that, I felt terrified of what she might go through if I didn't get better. That is, if she didn't leave first.

"Can you help me?" I asked, wiping my eyes and nose and face with my shirt. "Because I don't want to lose you. I can't lose you."

"I can try. But at the end of the day, you'll have to do this yourself. I think you know that."

"Yeah."

"Well, I don't really know where to begin, but I will call the doctor, okay? Maybe they have someone you can talk to."

"Okay. Anything. I'll start anywhere."

When we got home, she called the nurse hotline at the hospital. I sat right next to her, listening, as the nurse told her about the Chemical

Dependency Recovery Program, or CDRP. Outpatient rehab. Annie looked at me after the nurse finished. I nodded back to her, solemnly. They scheduled an intake appointment for the morning.

I knew I didn't want to lose Annie. I knew I didn't want to be this person anymore. I wanted to take some kind of step. But I was scared shitless because I didn't actually know what that step was. *Do I even really want to know? What if they say I have to quit? What am I gonna do if I hear that?* I was afraid to even imagine what I'd do without a drink in all those moments I needed one.

Because those moments—they were all the fucking time.

Part Eight

Chapter 1 - Paula

The next morning, Annie drove me to the CDRP. I told her she didn't need to take an hour off from work, but she insisted. I guessed she'd envisioned me driving myself there, staring at the front door for a while, and then getting the fuck out of dodge. So, instead, she dropped me off, parked the car, and didn't leave until she saw the front door shut behind me.

The place looked nothing like the main hospital building across the street, where everyone else went for their flu shots and annual checkups. A security guard manned the main entrance. At first, the big, burly bouncer seemed a bit over the top for a hospital department. But I quickly remembered everybody coming in here was some kind of addict—present company included.

In the lobby, most of the walls had chipped or peeling paint. I would have spotted more if not for the tattered, xeroxed fliers crudely stapled everywhere. The pink, blue, and yellow sheets fashioned a collage of upcoming meetings for Alcoholics Anonymous, Narcotics Anonymous, and Al-Anon.

When I got to the counter, a thick piece of glass separated me from the receptionist. As I slid my hospital membership card through a small hole, I wondered what might have happened to make them put it up. I pictured desperate people, in the throes of withdrawal, grabbing and clawing.

I sat down in the waiting room and picked up a *Car & Driver*. The cover featured the "brand-new" Camaro—the same one that had been on the road for a year. I tried a *Sports Illustrated* next, which I hoped was slightly more current. But the *SI* had February's Super Bowl-winning Steelers on the cover. It was July. I tossed both magazines back on the coffee table and slouched into my chair.

The receptionist gave a young woman a plastic receptacle for a drug test. The security guard stopped a screaming homeless man at the front door. A staff person rushed frantically down a corridor after a patient. The first woman came back from the restroom and gave the dark, dehydrated testing sample back to the receptionist through the little opening in the bulletproof glass. *Jesus. Where the fuck am I?*

I suddenly felt like I did the first few days at Butler, when I'd been resistant to acknowledge I belonged there. Reluctant to admit I hadn't just gotten off on the wrong floor by mistake. No, just like then, this wasn't a fluke. I was where I needed to be. I couldn't be shocked at anything or judgmental of anyone. We'd all gotten ourselves here, one way or another. At that, my eyes welled up with tears for the second time in as many days.

"David?" A bright, cheerful voice called out.

"Yep, that's me." I stood up and followed her down a hall.

Her office didn't look much better than the lobby. The paint hung on the wall for dear life. The sole window had rust around the metal edges. But despite the CDRP's maintenance budget, she cared about the space. Her bookshelf was organized perfectly with editions of the Diagnostic and Statistical Manual and other academic and topical books. She had plants, framed pictures, and a jar of candy for patients.

She even had a rug that she'd likely bought with her own funds to top the old, gray carpet.

"So, tell me why you're here," she said.

I didn't enjoy the obligatory, redundant recapitulations every time I met a new doctor or mental health professional. I knew they all had my file, after all. But I understood it wouldn't happen any other way. I started by telling her how much I drank in college. Then I told her about the manic and depressive episodes that started around the time I graduated. I told her I wanted to die on the Bay Bridge and for a couple of weeks after. I told her about my years in Rhode Island and getting diagnosed with bipolar disorder. Then I landed the plane at the present day—living in the hell of my deteriorated mental health and self-medication.

She just stared intently at me as I spoke, leaning forward in her seat, chin perched on two fists. She seemed so interested in what I said. Quite different from my meetings with Dr. Ewing. Despite all the chaos outside her little office, she made me feel like I was in a vacuum. I forgot about the homeless dude banging on the front door, the urine sample handed over in the lobby, and the expired subscription to *Car & Driver*.

"More and more, when I'm really drunk, I get so angry. So aggressive. A couple of cops approached me here in the city a while back, and I just lost my head. And it happened again recently in New Hampshire. I just always end up exploding."

"So, there wasn't always that aggression?"

"Right. It wasn't like that before."

"And when did that start, exactly?"

"Not until the last few years. After I moved back from Rhode Island. Around the same time as I was diagnosed bipolar and started taking medication."

"That may not be a coincidence, David," she says.

I know.

"Why don't you start by just coming to a group that I lead? It's called dual diagnosis. Mental illness and addiction. We meet every week, and there's one tonight. It would be great if you could join. No obligation. Just show up and see what you think."

"Uh—okay. But is everyone in the group sober?"

"No. Some are, and some aren't. It's not required."

"Okay, I'll come."

In some part, it was because she didn't tell me I had to stop drinking right away that I was quick to agree. And, also, I liked Paula. She was disarming and her empathy felt deep and genuine. I left her office with something in my pocket… a bit of hope for the future.

Chapter 2 - Moderation

That workday was long and the drive to the meeting at CDRP was painstaking. I didn't know what lay ahead. Alcohol had been a grave danger to me, but it offered me certainty in exchange. Certainty that the warm fire it started in my belly would come to subdue my nagging, invasive thoughts. What I wasn't certain of was whether I truly could trade that in, even if for my partner and my own well-being. Starting this program might force me to answer that very question.

I reminded myself that I didn't have to make a commitment, or even a plan, right away. That I would just go try a group that helped people manage addiction and mental illness. That it didn't have to be any more than that, yet. But I also reminded myself that I *did* have to do something *now*. Annie's words—*I can't wait forever*—still lingered in the air. More than alcohol, losing Annie, my other companion, was unthinkable. Without her I would surely plummet even farther down the hole I had dug. At those depths, I'd have no companion at all but booze and, of course, the animal. Who knew how long I could survive with just them.

I took a string of deep breaths after parking my car in the hospital garage. *A pull of whiskey could really help me get through this.* My mind immediately pinpointed the closest store. *Stop it. Be better than that.* After one more deep breath, I got out and shut the driver's side door. I passed the stoic bruiser of a security guard and quickly walked through the waiting room. I avoided meeting anyone's eyes. I had a fear of someone seeing my face and maybe forming a memory of me. I wanted to slip in and out like a ghost.

The room was virtually bare save a dozen folding seats. Some of the chairs were black, others gray, and a few brown. A threadbare ring worn deep into the carpet showed where they'd been arranged every few hours, every day, every week, for years. The walls had no decor—not even posters with cliched, motivational quotes. Just two, very small windows, which I imagined myself squirming through.

Paula greeted the group. "Welcome, everyone. This group is about understanding and addressing the dual diagnosis of addiction and mental illness." She continued with something like a premise, "Let me make clear that being sober or clean is not a requirement here. Moderation can be successful. But you're all encouraged to at least consider ways to move toward a sobriety-based treatment."

Sobriety-based treatment. It startled me a bit, even though I knew it was coming. I wanted to manage, moderate, and balance. But *sobriety-based treatment*—that sounded like finality. I just wanted to be like everyone else when they drank. To have some beers with friends and watch a game. To drink a couple of glasses of wine at dinner with Annie. Maybe even throw back a few shots if it was someone's birthday party. But to cut it out entirely? The ground trembled underneath my Jordans.

I watched everyone as we went around the circle and introduced ourselves. I was curious to know if they seemed nervous about being here, like me. Or if they seemed comfortable, like they'd done it plenty of times. One guy caught my attention right away. He had a smile on his face that would have been suitable for a fun networking mixer, not sitting in a circle of depressed addicts.

My eyes lingered for a few extra seconds on a young lady after her introduction. She looked like she was my age. And she looked nervous, too. Maybe she'd also wondered if she could crawl through one of the windows. She probably used to have more color in her skin, I thought. And perhaps she'd lost weight. Her body looked like it should have more fullness to it. *You're not a drinker—something else. Alcohol didn't do all this to you, did it?*

Paula started by asking people to share what brought them to the group. The guy with the out-of-place grin on his face quickly volunteered to speak first. I'd learned at Butler that there was usually someone in the group that wanted to use up all the room's oxygen. And, save for Larry, they usually grated on me. But they also provided good insurance against me getting nudged to speak before I was ready.

He shared very casually, with excitable inflection and gesticulation. "Well, I'm a regular, but I haven't been in a few weeks. So, anyways, I use coke. Too much. And I'm also manic depressive. I know, bad combo, right?! So, I was doing good and didn't do any for a couple of weeks. But then *laaast* weekend I went on a *huuuge* bender," he said. "I did way too much blow, and I cheated on my boyfriend again. And then we got into a fight, and now he wants to kick me out, but—"

Paula knew how to make sure *some* of the oxygen was left for the reticent ones. "Thanks for sharing. Let me get to some new folks. What motivated *you* to join us tonight?" She looked over at the young lady, who I'd silently made my companion for the evening.

Her eyes darted up from their fixation on the floor. "Umm, sorry, I wasn't really expecting to say anything."

"That's okay, take your time," Paula said, with a warm, earnest smile.

"Well, I've had depression for years and years, like, since I was young," she answered, quietly. "And then I started drinking in my twenties. Not a lot at first. Just to make stuff easier. Parties or dates or whatever. Things where there were people, honestly. It then got to where I was drinking almost every day."

It is booze, after all?

"I got a DUI a couple of weeks back, and it just freaked me out. A few years ago, I could have never imagined that happening to me. And now it didn't even seem like that big of a deal, and that feeling, of it being

—I don't know—just normal. It scared the shit out of me. And, so, here I am. I just need to fix this before it's too late."

Then Paula moved on to the next leading question. "So you are all here because you want to find ways to manage an illness and an addiction. Coming here tonight is courageous in itself, of course. But are there any other steps anyone has taken so far that you can share with us? David, how about you?"

Shit. I'm not the one to ask. I haven't taken any steps. I was just in jail like three days ago.

"I don't know," I quietly muttered. "I came tonight. That's it so far."

"And before you decided to come here?" she quickly volleyed back.

"Oh, well, I went to see you," I offered.

"Why did you come see me?" she pressed, refusing to let me off the hook.

"I don't know. I guess I've just been realizing how messed up things have gotten. It started a long time ago. I've never been able to control the drinking. And then I was diagnosed with bipolar, six or seven years ago. I take different meds and stuff, but I just really use alcohol, I guess, more than anything else." I was surprised at my honesty with total strangers. My eyes welled up at hearing myself say that out loud. *What the fuck, man. Keep it together.*

She didn't push me any farther. Maybe she looked at my eyes and saw the levee about to break. Or maybe she saw them thoroughly inspect the exit door. Whatever it was, she knew the right moment to stop. "Thank you for sharing, David. I'm glad you joined us here tonight."

After that, I couldn't hear the group. I could only hear my fears manifesting into sharp commands. *I don't need to quit yet, but I do need to figure out how to manage it. And figure out how to drink reasonable amounts. Like most people do. If quitting altogether is the only way, I don't know if I can do it. But I can make a plan to moderate, I think.*

I'll start with six drinks. That should be a lot. But it's not really anymore. I won't lose control at six. I'll just have to drink a lot slower. I can't be at six at eight fucking thirty. I'll go out a little later, so I don't get a head start. And I'll only get drinks when other people do, so I stay at everyone else's pace.

This will be good for me. My friends will like me more. I'll like me more. Most of all, Annie will like me more.

I had a plan, and one that fit into the context of the group. Paula would support it. I knew she wanted us all sober and clean eventually, but she didn't oppose moderation. I did need to cut back—*way* back—but I'd show Annie, my friends, and myself that I could be much better without going entirely sober.

My new plan had me energized. After the meeting, I decided to go for a run. I had all but given up on running. It had gotten too hard. My body was heavier and slower. My feet didn't pop up off the ground after each step and ping me along like they used to. When running had started to feel like I was fighting through something viscous, I'd taken up boxing.

As far as activities, boxing suited me best at the time. I could bring my nasty animal with me and let it snarl and gnash its teeth. I liked to give the heavy bags a face. My targets could be the goons I'd tumbled with or the cops that had trampled me. Or, on a grim, gloomy day, it could just be me, fighting what I saw in the mirror. I imagined heavy, booming punches denting my face, liver, and ribs.

Eventually, I got a boxing license so the targets could hit me back. I loved exchanging slugs back and forth with other young dudes. One guy broke my nose. I let it heal on its own, stupidly, and left it pointing about thirty degrees to the right. When I finally got it looked at, I found out it had been broken into five little pieces. I found a strange satisfaction in leaving it untended for months. A weird battle scar, perhaps. Or maybe a projection of the way I'd felt inside—very, very broken.

But the day after the CDRP meeting, I decided I would get back on the road again. I'd come to find the most solace in the test of endurance training during all those years of rowing. My knees and ankles churned reluctantly, like dry, dormant bicycle gears. But I pushed through the rust for about four miles. It wasn't pretty, and the speed from my early twenties was entirely gone. But it was four miles more than I'd run in a while. And I didn't break my nose during any of them. That run, on top of having a plan and some resolve to moderate drinking, was enough to make me feel victorious. I just had to stay the course.

Chapter 3 - Six Drinks and Six Strings

Most people didn't even get to six drinks in one night. Yet, that was my bare fucking minimum. Still, it was a huge step in the right direction. I got into the habit of counting my drinks, paying attention to how much time passed between them, and even measuring my sips so my drink could last longer. It took sustained focus throughout the night, like refusing to itch a gnarly mosquito bite. But it worked.

James' girlfriend threw him a birthday party that summer. Before Annie and I left our apartment, I steeled myself. *Six drinks, not one more. Kelsey already doesn't like you hanging around him—don't make it worse.* I got my first drink and slowly sipped it while doing some mental math. *I'll be out for about three hours. A hundred and eighty minutes divided by six drinks is a drink every half an hour. Or something like that. This is doable.*

"Dave, you getting another drink? Will you get me one when you go to the bar?" James asked, towards the end of dinner.

"Uh—not right now, actually. Gonna wait a bit longer. But yeah, I got you for sure."

"Ha! That's definitely not what I expected you to say! Good for you, bro. But can you go get mine now? Cause—you know—it's my birthday, dog."

"Sure." I smiled. "Do you want me to see if they also have a little birthday tiara you can wear?"

His recognition felt good. On the other hand, his initial, wide-eyed incredulity stung a bit. As I walked back from the bar with his drink, it occurred to me that I'd probably never left a bar without a drink for *me*. I liked the way that made me feel.

I visited Paula weekly and kept going to her dual diagnosis groups, too. I even kept my appointment with my psychiatrist, Dr. Ewing. I still wasn't warmed to him, but since I had to see him, I figured I'd tell him about my work with Paula at the CDRP. I thought the effort I made to manage drinking might pique his interest.

"How have you been, David?"

"Pretty good! I have some pretty good news. I actually started going to the Chemical Dependency Recovery Program."

"Oh, that's good. What prompted that?"

What do you think prompted it? "I've just been drinking too much. And—I don't think I've mentioned it to you—but I've been getting into trouble." I left space for him to ask me *what* trouble I was referring to, but he didn't. "And my girlfriend—my other friends probably, too—she's having a hard time with it. I'm putting her in a bad spot, and I don't want to end up pushing her away."

"Well, I think that's positive news. Have you found that drinking has made it harder to control or manage your bipolar symptoms?"

No fucking shit, Doc. "I imagine it hasn't helped."

He either didn't believe in me or he just didn't really care. It was a huge hospital—I knew he had a ton of patients. I assumed that he reserved his highest measure of dedication to the patients he saw trying the hardest to be successful in their treatment. Maybe my coldness towards him was just a response to feeling a bit rejected.

Until then, I'd always found some comfort in the cold space between his silly medicine ball chair and the couch. Disliking him had just been another excuse that I'd teed up for myself. But his indifference at this particular appointment nipped me a bit. I thought he might be more encouraging.

Annie saw my little nuggets of effort and tracked them closely. On Mondays, she knew whether I went to see Paula or not. On Tuesdays, she could tell if I'd gone to the dual-diagnosis group before I even told her. When we went out, she always knew how many drinks I'd had. I felt pride when she saw me slowly sip my drinks. It felt like doing well on a quiz in school.

We went on an anniversary dinner in the early fall. As we sat across from each other, I realized it had been a long time since I hadn't felt guilty when I looked at her. I knew I still had a long way to go, but the changes of the past few months had given me a foothold. Our conversation at dinner wasn't strained by my shame or her disappointment. Instead, we looked forward.

"What do you want to do for Christmas this year?" I asked.

"Let's get a rental in Tahoe and go skiing. Just the two of us."

"Great. What about family visits?"

"Let's tell each of our families that we're visiting the other, and then just disappear."

"I love it."

We went home after dinner and fell asleep in each other's arms. It felt like it used to when our future was open and bright. Before I put a cloud over it. For Annie, I wanted to be better. And sure—for myself, my job, my friends, all of that, too. But it was Annie that gave me the greatest desire to change.

I suddenly had more time. I spent fewer hours drinking or hung over. But more than just time availed— a *desire* surfaced. Desire to do more, to be more. I never lost the interest to work with kids after leaving Rhode Island. I just didn't have the capacity. I was consumed by benders or hangovers.

A friend of Annie's suggested a program called CASA—Court-Appointed Special Advocates—for foster children in the Bay Area. I signed up to get involved in no time. Volunteers mentored the kids and advocated on their behalf at custody hearings. Many of these kids had been taken out of their homes because of drugs, violence, or both. Foster placements were no picnic, either. Foster care often meant living in a group home with a dozen other kids packed into a small house with no supervision. The calculus often boiled down to just determining the lesser of two evils—life with the family or life at the group home.

During training, I sat amongst a bunch of high-achieving young adults looking to pad their already fat resumes, adding something wholesome for a law or business school application. I guess my resume wasn't out of place—Dartmouth and then two years in social work. Nonetheless, around this group, I felt decidedly like an imposter. A familiar feeling.

My first assignment was Isaiah. He was a sixteen-year-old from Hunter's Point, San Francisco's roughest neighborhood. His parents, both drug addicts, were losing custody of their kids. The first time I pulled up, Isaiah's mom started screaming at me from the front steps of their house. Past her, through the ajar front door, I saw piles of trash strewn throughout. His little brother stood quietly behind her as she cursed at me and scowled.

He was tough on me, at first. For a month or two of visits, I could barely get him to talk. He fixated on his phone, which didn't actually have service. It had some games—enough for him to tune me out. He resented the county and the courts getting in the middle of his family. And, by extension, he resented me, too.

But like with Brandon in Rhode Island, I didn't let up. I asked questions to fill the silence. *What's your favorite song right now? Do you like the Warriors? What would you pick if you could only eat one thing for the rest of your life?* It eventually wore him down. Pretty soon, he started giving answers. He liked Flo Rida way too much, didn't really give a shit about sports, and would happily eat pizza every day.

Once I got him talking to me, it didn't take long to find out he loved movies. I could work with that. He rarely got to go to the theater, so he didn't care what movie we saw. Before the movie, he'd load up on theater food. I pretended not to notice that he stuffed half of it in his pockets for when he got home.

I also found out he wanted to learn to play an instrument. He'd always liked music but had never taken so much as a piano lesson. I asked him what he'd learn if he could. He said he thought guitar was cool. Before our next visit, I bought him a used guitar and signed him up for six lessons. I wasn't supposed to do it—the program didn't allow any gifts more than twenty bucks. But it seemed like the only way he'd get one.

"Hey, Isaiah," I said as he got in the car. "Have a look in the back seat."

"What's this for?" he said, stunned, once he recognized the unmistakable shape of a guitar case.

"It's yours, man."

"What? Are you for real?"

"Yup. And you got some lessons already set up. You just gotta get yourself there and you gotta practice. That's it."

"Yo, this is some of the nicest shit anyone has done for me. Thank you. I'll take hella good care of it."

"Bet your ass."

Part Nine

Chapter 1 - New Balance

The reduction in hangovers gave me time to whip my ass back into shape. I'd forgotten how much I loved working out. I loved seeing the sweat from my face hit the floor. I loved pumping music until my ears rang. And I loved answering all the tough, gnarly questions that surfaced. *Can I fight the urge to stop? Can I keep going? Can I go even harder?* Boxing had become a satisfying and suitable new hobby. And I always relished a game or six of pick-up basketball. But running... running stirred up that hard-fought gratification I felt rowing on the Connecticut River, pushing myself through pain and fear.

Each week, I did several short runs after work and one long one on Saturday or Sunday. After a few months of drinking less and running more, I could run eight miles in an hour again. I even signed up for a half marathon in San Francisco. Training for the race gave me one more reason to stay measured with my drinking. And it served to remind me that I was quite capable of fighting through challenges, obstacles, and pain.

On top of all that, I remembered that alcohol wasn't the only thing that could get me drunk. The zippy buzz that lingered for a while after a long run or a grueling workout intoxicated me. There was nothing like surging through the last mile of a run, pulling up to a stop, and filling my lungs with huge plumes of clean, crisp air.

Before rowing, Will had been a cross-country runner. When he was in good condition, he was fast. Smoking fast. But he was out of shape like me. Thicker and slower from years of too many Bud heavies and Camel lights. But also like me, he'd been sniffing around for a reason to revive himself. He'd cut his own drinking back and wanted to take on his first fitness challenge, even if it was a big one. I wondered how much my own habit had exacerbated his binge-drinking. A lot, I reconciled, sadly.

"Hey, man!" I called him out of the blue one day after a good weekday jaunt. "So, I signed up for a half marathon in SF. You wanna do it with me?"

"Dave, do you know the last time I went for a run?"

"No, but I knew I needed a month's head start on training if I'm gonna keep up with you. So that's why I waited to call you until now."

"Ha! Jerk. Okay, fuck it. I'm in."

Over the next month, we talked every day or two about our workouts. A freeness spread through our conversations. I'd never stopped feeling terrible about getting him dragged to jail with me—it hung in the back of my mind whenever we talked. It was refreshing to have something innocent and clean to fill our talks with. Amazed, I watched how quickly he found his legs. Only a month after throwing up at the end of his first run, he was within striking distance of doing a half marathon in ninety minutes.

I made my last training run before the race an easy one. It was just an idyllic, almost relaxing, trot. For an hour, give or take, I felt at peace, and I thought about how much better my life was. I was happier, more productive, closer to Annie, and I was even uncovering an old, hibernating six-pack that I hadn't seen in years. *This is perfect. Don't fuck it up,* I reminded myself.

Poor Will couldn't get off from work on Friday, so he landed from Chicago the evening before the Saturday morning race.

"Sweet Prince! Over here!" I shouted from my idling car.

He trotted over with his bag and hopped in before I could pull over.

"Are you fired up, or what?" I asked him.

"Eh, we'll see. Ask me tomorrow morning. How about you?"

"I'm nervous, but, you know, in that good way."

"Same. I needed this. My ass was so out of shape!" he said. "Thanks for putting this together, by the way. You've been doing a lot better, bro, I'm happy for you."

"Yeah, man. I've been moderating a bit. It's been good." *A bit.* The hedge shot right out reflexively, as if I wanted to quickly set the record straight. I didn't want his expectations of me elevated too high. The moderation was uncharted territory for me. I didn't know how long it would last, and I didn't quite want anyone getting used to it. *What if I don't—or can't—keep this up?* The question lingered with every passing week.

We got home late and sank into *300,* my favorite graphic-novel-inspired, historical-semi-non-fiction film. When I heard Will snoring lightly on the couch, I put a blanket on him and popped his shoes off. I looked at him for a second. I was lucky to have him as my friend, I thought. He came for the race, sure, but really he came to support me. Hell, he might have even got himself in shape to run thirteen miles just to be a good friend. Not that many people would do that, would they? But I didn't know if I was worth all his effort. I felt scared I'd backslide, sooner or later, and let him and Annie down.

By the time I woke up the next morning, Will had already made us coffee and had started at least his second cup. "Let's do this!"

"Oh, wow," I said. "You don't sound anything like the whiny bitch I picked up at the airport last night. I have something for you." I grabbed a TJ Maxx shopping bag and pulled out two matching outfits—knee-high socks, tiny black shorts, little black vests that I took off a couple three-piece suits, and two paddy hats.

"That's what we're wearing?"

"Absolutely."

"Delightful."

We threw on our duds and laughed at one another. The vest was way too tight on Will. Meanwhile, the shorts were barely keeping me concealed. On cue, Annie walked into the living room.

"What in the world are you... nevermind, you look great."

We finished our coffee and piled into Annie's Jeep and drove to the start. Dawn was trying to break, but the air was dense and dark with trademark San Francisco fog. While the night and morning wrestled, the three of us hung around in Annie's car drinking coffee and listening to Will's gripes about his new, boring insurance job—which did indeed sound awfully banal—until the time came to funnel into the starting gate.

"Okay, boys. Good luck. See you at the finish."

"Babe, you don't have to pick us up. It was so nice of you to drop us off."

"Yeah, Annie, I'll drag your boyfriend's limp carcass home."

"I want to," Annie said. "I like seeing all the race hoopla. And, you know, I'm just happy you're doing this."

Her sentiment suddenly caused another reflex inside of me. It sounded more hopeful—expectant, even—than I was comfortable with, much like Will's comments on the way back from the airport. It had only been a couple of months since I started cutting back. And I still drank every week, after all, just not enough to black out. It was hardly anything to celebrate just yet, I thought, and I didn't want to be backed into a corner.

"Okay, time to hit it!" I blurted. "Babe, see you soon, this side or the other."

As soon as we popped out of the car, we got a few laughs and claps from other runners. If we didn't race well, at least we had one accolade to take home—best-dressed. Will started a bit before me. He was going out behind the ninety-minute pacesetter. Not me. I'd leave with the one hour and forty-minute pack. *Even with an extra month of training, this motherfucker is still gonna smoke me. Unbelievable.*

"Good luck, bro! Go get it!" I shouted as he took off down the Embarcadero. A minute later, it was my turn. I felt nervous but, just like all my long training runs, I thought, *One mile at a time.*

First mile marker. The piers. *I'm usually sleeping on the couch right about now. I'd have just stopped drinking a few hours ago.* I hadn't worked out that early since morning crew practices almost a decade before.

Second mile. Fisherman's Wharf. *This pace feels pretty good. And this air... the air is perfect.* I loved running in heavy fog. It reminded me of those mornings rowing when the mist hung over the calm, flat water.

Fourth mile. Palace of Fine Arts. *Great scene in* The Rock *right here, after Sean Connery steals the Hummer from the rich Euro guy.* The pace came easily and freely. I knew the ease wouldn't last, but I hoped I could squeeze a few more miles out of it before things got... uncomfortable.

Sixth mile. Golden Gate Bridge. *I always thought it was flat, no way. Fuckin' windy, too. But stop complaining.* The magnificence of the bridge *was* inspiring, even with sneaky elevation change and a stiff crosswind. The massive red towers and thick cables ascended into the fog, giving the appearance that they rose up for miles.

Ninth mile. Sea Cliff. *These hills are just as steep as the last ones. But they feel easier, somehow.* It was suddenly no longer dangerous to think about the finish line. It was a measurable, finite eventuality and no longer just a looming, murky possibility. The question was, how hard did I want to push myself down the stretch?

Eleventh mile. The Sunset District. *Just count down the avenues. From fortieth to nineteenth. One at a time, I can do that.* I tried to think of an athlete that wore the number of every avenue I passed on their jersey. *Twenty-one... Deion Sanders... Twenty... Gary Payton... Nineteen... Shit, who the hell wore nineteen?*

Thirteenth mile. *Are you going to choose courage right now? Take it up a notch. It's supposed to fucking hurt... Holy shit, is that Will? No fuckin' way. He's gassed. I could pass him... Not many chances to edge out Will in a footrace. No, I'll push him through it, like he'd do for me, and get us to the finish line together.*

I sided up next to Will and gave him a pat on the butt. He looked as tired as I'd ever seen him in all our years training together. Through the pain, though, he mustered a grin when he saw me. He found one more push, deep down in his guts, and we crossed the finish line together after charging through the last mile.

Will was toast. He sprawled out on the ground and closed his eyes, his chest heaving up and down. I still had a little adrenaline keeping me upright. While he sucked in wind, I walked off the burning lactic acid and looked for food and water. I grabbed six bottles of water, four greenish bananas, and two shiny participation medals.

I sat down next to him, relishing the electric buzz pinging through my body. I hadn't had anything to drink in a week. But it wasn't an achy seven days spent resisting a constant gravitational pull. No, something stood between the alcohol and me. In that space where yearning and need usually resided, I felt contentment instead. Joyfulness, even.

My time was a personal best by a long shot. One hour and thirty-seven minutes. Not bad, considering how rough I'd been on my body over the years—particularly on my insides. *What if I always worked this hard? I could be fast as hell. Fast enough to beat Will without sneaking up on him from behind? Probably not.*

"Guys, you made it!" Annie hollered as soon as she spotted us in the sea of tired, floppy people.

"Hi, babe! Yup, we did. Barely, though."

"How did it go?"

"It wasn't pretty, but we got through it." It was an understatement, but I didn't want to celebrate too openly.

"Oh, don't be modest," Will clapped back. "You killed it."

"Okay. I had a good run. *We* had a good run."

I stopped there, without conceding that the run was actually cathartic. A vindication of my soul that I desperately needed. I didn't know what I had to lose by being honest, but I couldn't quite let them see the full measure of emotion. Somewhere inside of me, perhaps, I knew that sooner or later, I might let them down, again.

When we got back to the apartment, at about nine a.m., Will went down immediately for a nap. I could have crashed hard, too, but I didn't want to let any time pass while I felt that good. I didn't know how long it could last. Annie and I sat outside on our little porch, sipping coffee that she'd brewed up for us.

"I'm proud of you, love."

"Thanks. I feel good about it. There was a rough patch around mile nine, but—"

"No, not your race. I don't care about that. I'm just proud of *you*."

"Thanks, love. Yeah, I haven't felt this good in a while."

Will and I stayed in that afternoon and night except for a trip to Barney's Hamburgers, a favorite in my neighborhood, for half-pound bacon cheeseburgers, mounds of curly fries, and milkshakes. Annie joined, though mostly just to hang with us and dabble in the curlies.

With the runner's high starting to fade, we played Scrabble and watched movies until we passed out. It was a good day.

Chapter 2 - Yes, Your Honor

My grandfather fought cancer for as long as any doctor had thought possible. He went round after round with chemotherapy and radiation at ninety years old and refused to go down. Eventually, pneumonia insidiously crept in and dealt the final blow. I sat at his side when he passed, along with my mom and the rest of our family. Even after his lungs could no longer gasp for air through the ventilator, his heart kept beating for several more minutes, unwilling to yield. He hadn't died young, but it was still devastating. I'd revered him since I was a kid.

He passed a few days before the court date I'd earned in New Hampshire. The situation made me feel awful. I should have been helping my mom with arrangements at home, but instead I would have to fly back to the East Coast to plead guilty to being a fucking idiot and an asshole.

A few days before my date, my public defender called me. He told me that if I plead, the court would drop the resisting arrest charge and just give me the misdemeanor for disorderly conduct.

"Okay, I see. Well, that sounds good, thank you," I said. "But is there any way I can do it from here?"

"I don't follow," he said.

"I mean, do I need to actually *go* to the courthouse? There's a funeral service for my grandfather."

He paused, probably wondering if I was joking. "Sorry for the loss," he said, flatly. "But, that's not how this works. Failure to appear means that they'll put a warrant out."

"Oh, okay. Got it." *Shit.*

I was happy with myself for cutting back the drinking and for working with Paula and going to dual diagnosis groups. But that self-satisfaction was met with waves of guilt, too. I could plainly see I'd become a lesser family member, a lesser partner to Annie, a lesser employee, a lesser… everything. I'd even been a lesser patient. I had a mental illness I hadn't been properly treating for years. Instead, I had been trying to drown it underneath a steady torrent of whiskey and beer. But the only person drowning was me.

Even now, a few days before the funeral, instead of being where I needed to be—with my family—I was stuck cleaning up a mess I had made months before. And I couldn't even tell them where I was going. I asked Annie to lie for me in case they reached out to ask. I planned to just disappear for a few days, with no explanation offered. But she said she wouldn't, so I just had to hope they didn't call.

On the plane to New Hampshire, I sat trapped—stuck reflecting on the dark reality I'd created over the past few years. I finally drank less, sure, but that gave me a clear view of just how sick I'd gotten. Throughout the flight, I noticed my distorted reflection from the little headrest TV staring back at me. I could do nothing to get out of my own sight.

New Hampshire was as remarkable as ever. The fall months were truly spectacular. I wished I was there for some other reason, like the annual August run to the summit of Mount Moosilauke that my team used to do. It was the highest peak for miles and miles. I remembered the exhaustion from booking it up the mountain under an intense sun. But I remembered the exhilaration, too, from seeing the blitz of yellow, orange, and red trees visible in every direction.

I stayed in the cheapest motel I could find. I rented a car, using the same calculus. I wanted no memory of this embarrassing trip, so the less I could put on my credit card statement, the less it would agitate me when I paid it in a couple weeks.

I felt anxious and couldn't sleep. *A drink would help me pass out right now. No, no, no, don't give in. I need to fall asleep on my own.* Eventually, after three cycles of the same SportsCenter episode, I drifted off.

It was already sweltering when I got to court, nearly ninety degrees by eight a.m. Other than the sweat bleeding through my white shirt, I looked pretty decent. I'd make a good impression on the judge, I figured. But once I scanned the courthouse lobby, I realized I could have dressed way, way down.

Aside from the attorneys, I was the only one wearing a suit. I looked around to see jeans, t-shirts, and even pajamas on one young woman who waited with her two kids. I saw Dunkin' coffee cups, *Guns & Ammo* magazines, and even chewing tobacco in the mouth of one old man. When the big doors to the courtroom opened, the defendants piled in and grabbed seats on long benches that looked like church pews. Cases were called based on an order I couldn't seem to figure out. I watched and listened intently to each one before me. I reminded myself not to silently judge anyone. *I'm here with them, and not by accident. We all fucked up. The only thing different about me is that I saw the dress code.*

The old man with the Copenhagen didn't remove the huge swab from his cheek when he stood up. A few shards of it had even driveled their way down to his jaw. It looked like little ants crawling on his face. His eyes looked absent. His body was old and frail and hollowed out. He was arrested for possession and DWI after crashing into a guardrail on the wrong side of the road. He had drifted off, high on Oxycontin, and veered into the oncoming lane.

He took his plea deal and left the courthouse alone. I thought he would be leaving with the sheriff and going to prison. Before he left, the judge shook his head and said to him, "Sir, I need you to be careful. You are going to get yourself or someone else killed."

I was surprised by how gentle the judge was with him. But so be it. I wanted to remain empathetic—just so long as I got nowhere near the old-timer on the highway.

The woman with the pajama bottoms followed. She had a small boy tucked under her arm and toted another around by his little wrist. She'd been arrested for a DUI while she was driving with a suspended license. After another lenient plea deal was recited, the judge added, "I hope that this event can teach you what's at stake for you and your children. Good luck."

After a bundle of DUIs, a handful of possessions, and one grand theft auto, the bailiff finally called my name. My public defender motioned for me to come up. My suit, even if a little wrinkled and fairly sweaty, still looked sharp. *I hope he can see I'm trying to get my shit together.*

As I stood there with my hands clasped in front of me, I thought of Isaiah. *I sit in those courtrooms at the same table as his lawyer and social worker. If only they could see me here.* I felt ashamed—and glad this courtroom was three thousand miles away.

"State your name," the bailiff said.

I introduced myself while trying to hold eye contact with the judge. It was like looking into a bright light, though. His gaze was well-practiced and intimidating. I took an oath and solemnly swore to tell the whole truth. While I recited, the judge looked down and quickly reviewed the file in front of him. Given how easy he was with the other defendants, I presumed that I would glide right through.

My attorney, now on his eleventh or twelfth case of the morning, quickly proposed the plea deal that had already been lobbed out in advance by the prosecutor. The judge finally looked up from the file, removed his glasses, and glared at me. He narrowed his eyes, craned his neck forward, and cocked his head at a slight angle. He had perfected the look. My head dropped, involuntarily. Bad dog.

Finally, he asks, "What do you do for a living, David?"

Why is he asking me about my job? "Uh—I do commercial real estate," I stammered.

He didn't reply.

The silence gave me the misguided urge to say something else. "My last job was social work. I still volunteer as a mentor—" *Why am I still rambling?*

"You work with kids?" he asked, suspiciously.

Shit. Bad start. He was about to dress me down. I could feel it. It was almost as if he had saved up all his scorn just for me. "Yes, Your

Honor, I do." I tried to pick my body up a bit and sound proud when I said it.

"That's concerning," he said.

I froze with a big lump in my throat.

After a long pause, he continued, "Do you think you're a good role model for the kids you work with?"

The lump got bigger as the rhetorical question cut deep. I didn't see it coming. I thought my Dartmouth diploma and my real estate gig and community service would have given me some extra points. Nope—he chastised me worse than anyone. Perhaps in spite of those things.

He waited for me to respond. *Oh, come on, man—are you really going to make me answer?* "I think—well, sir—Your Honor, I mean—I think people make mistakes."

"Okay. Well, I think you better *stop* making mistakes," he says. "Or those kids might be better off with someone else."

He read off the sentencing—a thousand bucks and a misdemeanor conviction. I was escorted out of the courtroom and shown where to make my thousand-dollar remittance. All the work I'd done to get my shit together suddenly felt trivial. Instead of feeling like I'd come a long way, I felt frustrated, like it was all for naught.

The lady at the booth cheerfully asked, "Would you like to pay with cash, check, or credit card?"

I handed her one card. "Credit card, please."

I handed her another. "Oh, wait—actually, can you split it?"

Chapter 3 - My Grandfather's Blood

It played in a loop in my head on the way to the airport. *Do you think you're a good role model for the kids you work with?* I thought of the weekend trips in college that I had skipped because I had an appointment to go jogging around the track with Gary. I thought of the guitar lessons and the brand-new guitar I got for Isaiah. And, of course, I thought of the couple of years that I spent with the juveniles in the woods of Rhode Island, where axes and rocks on occasion whizzed by my head.

I still felt the hot, burning blood shooting through my arms and legs by the time I got back on the plane. *I know I've screwed up, but I'm fucking college-educated, gainfully employed, and even volunteering on the side. And I had a goddamned shirt and motherfucking tie on in court.*

But it was just my own defiance and petulance fighting back. The judge wasn't wrong at all. He saw right through me in one five-minute hearing. I wanted to project my anger outward—at him, at the police, at anyone that didn't know the *real me*—but it was fraudulent, misguided blame. I wanted to believe that people knew I wasn't actually some alcoholic maniac. But it hit me that day. *Why would I be something other than what my actions and behaviors have shown them every night? That's all they've seen, for years. Maybe the damage is already done?*

I'd been so oblivious to something so obvious to everyone else. For years, I had convinced myself that my drinking wasn't a huge problem. Better yet, I'd convinced myself that no one *else* thought my drinking was a huge problem, either. In that moment, squeezed into a middle seat on coach, I felt a sudden and sharp humiliation.

My eyes opened to exactly what everyone else had already seen. The reckless binging, fighting, and arrests. The belligerence, anger, and impetuosity. I could see it all through others' eyes, stripped away from the excuses and promises. I was overwhelmed with a fear that I'd done too much to ever reclaim myself in their eyes—or my own. What if there was already a permanence to whom I had become? Would the past few months of moderation even make a dent in the way people saw me? Or had I carved a scar I could never erase? If so, what was the point of continuing to try? What if being a full-blown alcoholic forever is just… inevitable? My belief in myself, at that moment, was utterly non-existent.

And then, at a time I could have used some extra space and solitude, I had none. I sat squeezed between two hefty Southwest Airlines passengers and could feel both of their shoulders and forearms pressing into me. It was too much.

I could just fucking explode. I need to get out. I want to shove one of them into the window and chuck the other into the aisle. Then I want to run to the emergency escape door and kick it open. I'd hurl myself through the hatch, spread my arms and legs wide, and float through the sky. Like a Tom Cruise stunt from Mission Impossible. *But with no parachute.*

Fuck it. I need a little something. Now. I would stay under my limit, if not for discipline, at least on account of the outrageous cost of a tiny whiskey bottle. I pressed the button on the ceiling, even though I hated when other people did that. I ordered two little Jacks with Diet Coke. Enough to just calm the fuck down. The memorial service was tomorrow, and I still needed to write something to say.

It was a hundred and something degrees in Sacramento. I'd gone from one side of the country to the other, yet I could not escape the fucking heat. All five of us crammed into one stuffy car—my parents in front, and my sisters and I in the back. I squeezed into the middle, with my black pants glued to my legs and my white shirt fixed to my back. I forgot to take my jacket off before we piled in. I sat still, slowly melting.

I couldn't remember the last time the five of us were in such close quarters. I could see my mom's grief for her father in the corner of her eye, revealing itself around the edge of her dark sunglasses. I had a hard time looking at her, even from the back seat. It made me feel guilty.

"How are you holding up, mom?" My little sister broke the taut silence.

"It's really hard. But I'm okay, thank you. I'm glad we're all together right now. And you've all been so thoughtful these past few days."

"I'm glad we're all together, too," said my older sister.

The more we spoke, the car got hotter and stuffier. I felt like I was in an interrogation room waiting to be shaken down, with a bright, burning light in my face. But they weren't even thinking about me. It was just my own shame, screaming to get out.

The crowd was large. He had been a brigadier general in the Marines and had amassed a large, esteemed community around him. There were a handful of speakers including me. My grandmother had asked me to say something, knowing how much I loved him. I felt nervous. Nervous because public speaking makes people nervous. But also, nervous because I'd written my speech on a fucking airplane, last-minute after a couple of little six-dollar bottles of whiskey.

When my turn came, I stood up and introduced myself to the large audience. I was completely sober. As much as I would have liked to take the nervous edge off with a couple drinks, I would have felt too guilty drinking beforehand. The faces I saw spanned decades. I read to men and women of his generation, survivors of tragedies and triumphs, like the Great Depression and the two World Wars. I read to his children, witnesses of his greatness as a man, though also of his demons and his drinking and his anger. And I read to his grandchildren, kin that knew him in large part from stories told by our grandmother at family dinners. Because he never told his own.

I spoke of his influence on me and the lesson I'd learned: pursue everything you do with conviction. By the time I closed with a final paragraph, I saw tears running down the faces in the crowd. I took a pause as planned—and because I needed one to keep my own tears in check—then took a deep breath before continuing.

> *I can only hope that I have learned from him what I could. I can only hope that, like him, I choose courage over idleness in the years ahead of me. I hope there is some of his fight in me. That same fight that thwarted our nation's enemies and battled cancer for as long as possible. My middle name is his. But more than his name, I hope I have some of his blood in me, too. For his is the stuff that can make me better than I am, or than I thought I could be.*

People were clapping. I didn't expect clapping at a memorial. I was glad it reached out and touched people. But I was distraught. I felt like I was living a lie. What kind of grandson was I, I thought, and what would he have thought if he'd seen me yesterday? If only I was half the person he was. Shit, if only we were all half the person that he was. But I wasn't, I confessed to myself. I was smart like him, but my brain had been too drunk and absent to make good use of it. I was strong like him, but what if I didn't have the strength to ultimately win the fight against this addiction and the thirsty, relentless animal inside me?

We retreated to my grandparents' home for the wake. Most people filled glasses with alcohol. I watched the amber liquor rise to the top of my own glass, then took my whiskey to one of my grandfather's chairs and sat alone. People came up to tell me they appreciated what I said in my speech. With a look and a raise of my glass, I invited them to sit down next to me and breathe in the rich, distinguished air in my grandfather's home. *Let's collapse together into this old leather, give way to the grief, and let this whiskey relieve us.* Most just took a perfunctory sip and let me be while I got loaded.

I knew drowning the pain wasn't the right way to deal with the grief of that day, but I chucked my six-drink rule to the side. *I'll be back on track tomorrow, I promise. But tonight—fuck it.* I drank throughout the night, too morose to care about any silent reproach by my family. They could only watch me slowly sink into that chair until I fell asleep.

Part Ten

Chapter 1 - The Whale

In the days after my grandfather's memorial, I snapped myself back in line. I'd had a shitty few weeks—the memorial, the fucking court date, and a lot of taking inventory of just how far I'd fallen over the past few years. It all brought me close to just saying, *To hell with six drinks. I will black out as I fucking please.* But I challenged myself to fight off those impulses.

Each week I didn't get wasted gave me another shot of belief that I could learn to moderate and, hopefully, never have to just abstain from alcohol. This time around, I didn't start drinking more when I felt like I had things under control. But I never stopped wanting to feel the escape that alcohol gave me. So, I started finding highs a different way.

I knew how tenuous my mental health was. I'd already been playing with fire for years by drinking so much. So I always remembered to take my pills each morning, even in the midst of head-rattling hangovers. The medication worked, and I understood that it was probably all that stood between me and the psychiatric hospital, or worse. It was a matter of survival. But the allure of feeling high was relentless.

At first, I told myself I skipped the meds just to see if I still even needed them anymore–as if, maybe after years of a steady regimen of tablets and capsules, bipolar disorder magically disappeared. It only took a couple days for some familiar feelings of my unmedicated self to reemerge. I quickly recalled the sensations, but only the ones that I liked. I felt the fun, flowing energy again—that same mania that motored me through phases of my early twenties. But also, the same energy that always eventually screeched to a halt and revealed its dark, sinister counterpart.

One week, I kept the pills in the medicine cabinet untouched for the whole seven days. It was reckless and wild. But I let the idea seep into my head that if I wasn't drinking in excess, I wouldn't trigger any depressive episodes. I wanted so badly to experience an altered state that, if I couldn't get enough of it from alcohol, I'd even chase the deceptive high that came from skipping my mood stabilizers. It was an exhilarating buzz. Mania feels like an out-of-body experience. It made my extremities tingle all day, like an everlasting nicotine zing. I could run and jump and play for longer, as if my engine was supercharged. And, most of all, my guilt and shame temporarily gave way to waves of optimism and acuity.

I went into the next weekend on skates. The sky looked blue and bright. Blake, who hadn't yet gone to rehab, signed us up for a scavenger hunt foot race. It was an annual fundraising event for a charity. A couple hundred teams of two were given the same list of locations and landmarks. Some were conveniently conspicuous and some were outright obscure. We had to find them all and snap a photo. It sounded perfect to me. I was in great running shape following the half marathon, and I knew the city like the back of my hand. The race started at a bar in downtown SF. We parked Blake's car nearby and trotted over, sizing up the other teams piling in.

"We should smoke all these jokers!" Blake was eager.

"Man, is there a prize for this thing for when we dust everyone?" I asked, hoping we could score a couple gift cards at least.

"It's for charity, dude. I don't think there are prizes," Blake quipped back.

"What? Charity events definitely have prizes?"

"Oh, yeah." Blake slowly let out a breath. "Okay, maybe. Whatever it is, let's win it!"

The lists were handed out in envelopes and a party-store foghorn signaled when we could open them up and start charting our course. Blake was a cross-country skier in college and had great endurance. He wasn't as fast as Will, but he could keep a solid pace for about ten miles or more if a few of the harder clues led us astray.

We were off. It was a gorgeous day. The fog usually shrouding the San Francisco waterfront had lifted. Without my medicine tempering the arcing pendulum swings of my mood, the radiant energy from the sun turned into electricity in my body. I bounded through the streets, jogging in place every few blocks to wait for Blake to catch up. We bounced around the city, stopping to get pictures of ourselves at Coit Tower, Pier 39, Ghirardelli Square, and even in front of a mural of a whale that adorned the side of one of San Francisco's more infamous strip clubs. After we knocked every place off the list, we scurried our way back to the bar for a first-place finish. It turned out there *was* a prize for the winners—free lunch.

As we ate our celebratory meal, the trademark San Francisco fog returned. The bright and cheerful sky suddenly turned to its customary gray hue. And, as if I were in lockstep with the weather, I suddenly felt covered in a familiar shroud of gray as well. It set in without warning. Just the devilish flip of a switch.

"What's up, dude? You all right?" Blake asked as we walked back to his Tacoma after lunch. "You haven't said anything in a while."

"Huh? Oh, yeah. I don't know. Just started feeling weird."

"What kind of weird?" Blake didn't know I was bipolar, let alone playing with my medicine as of late.

"Just like... kinda sad."

"Well, do you want to get a few more beers?"

While Blake didn't know about my struggles with bipolar, he *did* know I was trying to cut back on alcohol. But he was a heavy drinker and a heavy user himself, and it seemed to me that he cared more about having a drinking companion than having a friend in good health. I could empathize, so his selfish offer didn't make me angry. I had the same impulses when I saw Will starting to reel his drinking in.

"No. It's way too early. If I get started now, I'll get carried away. Especially when I'm feeling off... like this."

Usually, alcohol would be the self-medication of choice if I felt depressed. But I'd made enough headway to resist the temptation to start drinking at noon, especially without mood stabilizers percolating in my brain. I just wanted to get home, take my pills, and try to sleep off the scary haze fomenting, before it took a stronger hold.

"For sure. Well, I've got a few Vicodin in the truck, too, if you want."

I knew better. But *knowing better* doesn't mean anything to addicts. I grabbed them, despite knowing better, for a few reasons. I *deserved* them because I'd cut back on drinking. I *needed* them because my meds might need a couple days to set in. And I *wanted* them... just fucking because. I'd spent months training myself to moderate my drinking. It took constant work and preparation. But I hadn't given painkillers the same effort, and I didn't have my guard up when they were thrust into my face.

"Maybe, yeah, okay. Just in case." *Yeah, just in case.*

I rushed into the bathroom when I got home and took my doses—300 milligrams of Lamictal, a mood stabilizer, and 200 milligrams of Zoloft, an antidepressant. I visualized the little particles of whatever zipping through my bloodstream and up into my brain, where they'd gently wind me down. I put the small handful of Vicodin Blake gave me in one of my med bottles. They were long, white pills, mixed in with the yellow Zoloft. I'd be fine and wouldn't need them, I thought. But knowing they were there made me feel safer.

Chapter 2 - Doritos, Hot Pockets, and Vicodin

A few days passed, and the swirling gray fog still hadn't lifted. By Tuesday, intrusive thoughts peppered my mind, hitting from all directions. The same unchecked images and impulses that terrorized me during the worst episodes were back with a vengeance. Cars that whooshed by me on the street exerted a magnetic pull, urging me to jump in their path. Open windows made me wonder what it would look like if my body flew out and cratered into the pavement. If a person stood too close to me, I pictured them without an ear or arm or head.

By Wednesday, even with my medicine back in me, the thoughts and feelings of despair hadn't subsided. The appearance of normalcy I'd been trying to hold up had given way. At home, I'd been hiding behind whatever sporting event was on TV, keeping our dialogue short. But by the middle of the week, Annie knew something was wrong. She knew the signs—a perceptible vacancy in my eyes or a subtle, intermittent grinding of my teeth.

"Are you doing okay?" she asked that evening, after we'd both gotten home from work. "You seem a bit far away."

"Yeah. I'm struggling some, actually."

"What's wrong?"

"I don't know, just feeling out of sorts."

"Sorry, love. Is it pretty bad?"

"Nah, not too bad. Just feeling a little bit down." That was the first lie.

"Did something happen to trigger it?"

"I'm not sure, it just comes and goes sometimes, you know." Then came the second.

"Have you been taking your medication?"

"Yeah. I miss a day once in a while, but that's all." Hat trick.

"Okay. And—" she paused, as if scared of what the answer might be. "What about the drinking?"

"I haven't had anything to drink since I first started feeling this way, actually." At least that part was true. "I know I need to figure out how to get through it without alcohol."

"That's good, I'm proud of you for that. Let me know how I can help."

"Thanks, love. I will. I'll be okay, it just needs to pass."

But I didn't know if it would pass. In the middle of an episode, no matter how many have come and gone before it, each has the most persuasive impression of permanence. *This feels too real. This time, I'm actually losing my mind.*

Annie finally left the room, too tired to keep me company while I stared absently at the wall. I was glad when she left. My intrusive thoughts turned onto her, filling my mind with bizarre and ghastly pictures of her as she sat a few feet away on the couch. I sat there, wondering if I might suddenly be taken over by an impulse to strangle her, like Patrick Bateman from *American-Psycho*.

About an hour later, my eyes still trained on ESPN, but my mind whirred frantically behind them. I was no closer to falling asleep. A Vicodin would help me pass out, I thought, and maybe fast forward me eight hours closer to restoring sanity. If not, it could at least numb the pain for a while. I crept into the bathroom and turned on the sink. Cloaked by the hissing sound of the running water, I fished out one of the 10 mg white oval pills from my bottle of yellow Zoloft and swallowed it down. Ten minutes later, my mind finally exhaled the haunting images and pervasive despair. I sunk into a deep sleep on the couch, temporarily shrouded in tranquility.

When I woke up, a vague numbness floated through me. I hadn't gotten drunk, I figured, so I shouldn't feel too bad. But within a couple of hours, scattered stings of guilt and anxiety began rattling through me. I meandered through menial tasks at work, unable to focus. By the time I got home, I felt no less distraught than the night before. I took another Vicodin, this time, with much less trepidation.

Blake had only given me three of them in the first place, so what was the harm? I'd mute the depression for a few days while it ran its course. By the time I ran out of pills, hopefully the depression would have released its grip. I took the third pill on Friday night. I even had a beer with it, feeling vindicated because it was the last one.

But I didn't feel better the next day. The episode hadn't run its course. Not at all. If my mood stabilizers and antidepressants were going to extinguish the flame, they were taking their sweet fucking time. Unfettered and unfiltered thoughts still zig-zagged through my head. But now, one thought emerged above the noise and calmed me in its clarity—taking more Vicodin would make me feel better.

It wasn't hard to convince myself that I wouldn't make a habit of it. *I just need a small bottle of my own to help me get through another week. I won't get more after that. And it isn't alcohol. I have problems with alcohol, but I don't have problems with pills. Why shouldn't I get myself what I need to feel better?* The reasons were fucking abundant, of course. But there was no better liar than my ill, addicted mind. And nothing more believable than my own bullshit. I sent a text to Blake and got his guy's number.

Fucking Tyler. He owned a liquor store near Blake's apartment, which we patronized often. He sold booze to private school kids for a markup and ran his own prescription drug retail business right from behind the counter. His store was in a nice neighborhood, so he was off the cops' radar. He'd carved out a nice little market share for himself—booze, Doritos, pills, and Hot Pockets.

It seemed like a strange line to cross. Popping a pill here and there because someone happened to have them was nothing. Commonplace. A fun little surprise for a Saturday night. But calling up a dealer to get my own felt different. I hadn't done that since buying weed in high school. I felt guilt but also excitement. Before I wrote Tyler a text, I justified it to myself again. *I'm in an episode. I can't fucking think straight. My thoughts are intrusive and scary. My medication isn't working quickly enough. The Vicodin will just help catch my fall.* And, of course, *I won't get any more after this.* That was sufficient reasoning, I decided.

Yo whatsup it's Dave. Blake's boy. Can I pick up something from the store?

For sure bro. Come thru tonight. How many.

Twenty, if u got it?

Aight c u later.

After work, I headed over to his store. Even though I had met Tyler dozens of times, I felt shy and insecure this time around. Not unlike the way I felt at the supermarket when I was a kid, asking people to buy me and Peter some Smirnoff. I walked in, hoping no one else was in the store to see me. But it was just Tyler, sporting a flat brim SF Giants hat and a sly grin as he leaned back against the counter and typed out a text on his phone.

"Hey, man," I said, a bit under my breath.

He looked up from his phone and gave me a big, charming smile. "Yo, Dave! What's up, dog? How you been?"

"You know, always good."

"Haha, aight. Yo, Blake told me y'all did a scavenger hunt. That's hella funny, bro! Man, y'all cats is always up to some shit."

"Uh huh. Won it, too." I didn't like that he knew anything particular about me, even my participation in a scavenger hunt.

"Nice, bro. All right, then, what's good?"

I dapped him up again, this time with a clump of twenties in my palm. He pulled a green pill bottle out of his pocket and slyly dropped it in my other hand. Then I bought a bag of Doritos Cool Ranch and a Diet Coke so I had something to leave with. As I walked back to my car, the awkwardness and ambivalence subsided. I had a sure-fire way to feel better, and it was only moments away. Nothing else mattered.

Those first few minutes—when the opioids just start to hit those ready and willing receptors—were sheer bliss. I felt warmth in the cold. Calm in the frenzy. A shield went up around me, fending off unwanted, unwelcome thoughts. They ricocheted off me like little BB's fired at a tank. To someone in a depressive episode, opioids, like alcohol, can be a force of gravity. They could deliver sanctum from those excruciating, menacing thoughts. And they could deliver a deep, immersive happiness, even if it was illusory.

I succumbed to my self-medication plan, giving myself a dose whenever I felt like it. The guilt I felt for taking the pills, after all the work I'd been doing to curb my drinking and seek treatment from the CDRP, easily dissipated in the haze. The week went by in a blur, not unlike the days at Butler, in a medicated, catatonic state.

I knew this was wild and reckless. I knew I could probably get hooked on the pills, just like Blake. I knew there was no kind of suitable alternative to alcohol. I knew Annie would recoil if she knew what I was doing. I *knew* these things. But that was just logic. And logic didn't stand a chance against the self-delusion of an addict.

Falling off the wagon. Regressing. I've always wondered what it looks like to people of the non-addicted, unafflicted persuasion. Do they think we're weak, lazy, and selfish? Do they stare and judge silently: *How could you? What were you thinking? Why would you throw away all the progress you made?* Sure, as if it were so rudimentary.

I was in pain. Writhing and twisting. Plagued by bizarre visions of blood and wreckage and suffocation. Drowning myself in alcohol again looked like a reprieve amid a storm. It was an illusion, of course. Just a desert mirage to a thirsty, emaciated wanderer. But I saw relief from agony and believed it was safe to touch. At least for a moment.

Chapter 3 - Two Steps Back

Earlier in the year, Alex got engaged to his college girlfriend. They'd planned an engagement party right before the holidays. The night before the party, I went out with a few friends who were already in town for the bash. I left the house high on Vicodin, and I planned to do just a little bit of drinking, well within the six-drink limit.

I wish I could have touched my fingers together, stopped time, and taken an unbiased moment to consider my options. A fork in the road, with Annie, Will, Paula, my CASA kids, and fun footraces to my left. Or, to my right, true despair. If only it worked that way. Instead, in a fog of drugs and alcohol and depression, I only saw a moment of relief in a flurry of whiskey shots.

The opioids and alcohol together, along with my medication, turned me upside down. I stopped counting after the first drink. Or, never counted at all. Before long, I picked a fight with a friend of the host. The animal, who'd been suppressed for months, relished its return. I left, embarrassed and angry, then went to some bars to drink alone. As angry as the host and other guests were at me, I was far angrier at myself. I'd slipped up, big time. *That guy* was on full display. It was like he never left. I drank myself stupid until I had blotted out whatever memory I had of embarrassing myself.

I woke up early the next morning and stuffed my face into my hands. I knew I'd fucked up. With my eyes squeezed tight, I looked through the darkness for memories. But it was a muddled blur. No distinct lines. Mixing pills and alcohol together made blacking out so easy. If I was just drinking, the memory loss was slower and proportional. Ten drinks—three-quarters memory. Fifteen drinks—half memory. And so on, linear. But there was no clear formula for me if I drank and popped pills. I was there one minute and gone the next.

What did I get into that argument about at that house party? Where did I go after? How the fuck did I get home? At that, I saw a shutter-speed image of myself lying on top of a parked car on a busy street and calling Annie for a ride home. After she, and then a few more people, didn't answer, Annie's best friend, Jane, had agreed to pick me up.

Without her usual patience and diplomacy, Annie darted her words at me from the doorway of the kitchen. "Why the hell would you call Jane!"

"Sorry. I just—I woke up on the hood of a car freaked out. I didn't know how I got there or where I was and just started calling people."

"Well, don't call *her*. Don't call any of my fucking friends and bring them into your shit. It's embarrassing! And then you acted like an ass in the car!"

"I did?" I scanned for memories of the ride home. Nothing. "What do you mean?"

"You packed a dip in the car and spit on the floor. What the fuck, man?"

Jesus. I'm fucking gross. "I'm so sorry. I didn't mean to. I'll call her and apologize. I drank way too much."

"And how much is that? Do you even know? I doubt it. And, no, don't call her. Just leave her alone."

"Okay. Sorry. More than six, I assume. Probably a lot more."

"What is happening? You were doing good."

"I know. I fucked up."

"I can't go backwards with you. I won't do it."

She had been a lot of things before. Distraught, consoling, helpful, empathetic. But she had never been so mad. So exasperated and out of patience. I had been toeing the line. But I didn't let myself realize just how closely.

Chapter 4 - Always Faithful

I felt like shit when I got to Alex's on the night of his engagement party. I looked like shit, too, wearing shitty jeans and a shitty cut-off t-shirt. My outside matched the inside. Annie didn't come with me. "No chance," was her exact response.

Alan and Carl, two of our good friends from Dartmouth, came over to join Alex and me. Alan played lacrosse with Alex. Carl was a star on the soccer team. I hadn't seen either of them in a couple of years, and I didn't want them to see me at my worst. I was close to tumbling all the way back down the hill I had just started climbing.

And if there was a moment to get my drink limit firmly reinstated, this was this one, because I knew Jake would be at the party. Alex had pegged both me and another friend of his, Jake, to be the best men in his wedding. I wished he had just chosen one of us, even if it was him. I didn't care. I just didn't want to stand there next to someone whose guts I detested so much.

"Look, I've said this like ten times already, every time you bring this up. He was my best friend throughout my entire childhood. He was loyal to me. More than anyone else."

"Aw, that's cute."

"Fuck off."

"I'm kidding, please finish."

"And then he joined the Marines. When there was a war going on, too. None of us did that. And that's just something that's admirable to me. No matter what."

"I know, bro, I know. But he's just said and done some awful shit, man." As soon as I said that, I knew I'd left myself extremely vulnerable to a counterpunch. *Oh, and you haven't?* "But hey, that's really loyal and thoughtful of you, though. I can appreciate that."

"I think being in combat probably messed him up some."

He was a fucking asshole long before he ever went to the Middle East. "Sure, I hear that," I said begrudgingly.

"Just don't start shit with him tonight. And don't get too fucked up."

A few years prior, when we were still in school, the three of us hung out over a winter break. Alex had hoped that his best friend from childhood and his college counterpart would get along. I went along with it. We'd lift some weights together or drink some beers. Maybe both, if I could stand listening to Jake's obnoxious diatribes for that long. He ranted about the teachers at his school treating white kids unfairly and the girls being stuck up, as if that was why he couldn't get one. Sufferable, barely, only for Alex's sake.

But then, everything changed. We ran into each other in the winter of 2001, a few months removed from the World Trade Center attack, at a party some old high school friends threw. When I went to bump his fist and briefly say hello, he didn't raise his hand to meet mine. Instead, he just looked at me, stepped inside my space, and said, "Do you know where your fucking cousins are? Because we're looking for them and are gonna kill their asses."

"What the fuck did you just say to me?"

Immediately, Alex stepped in between us and then corralled me outside.

"What the fuck are you doing, Alex? Did you hear what the fuck he just said?"

"I know, man. But you're the reasonable one, and you know it's not worth it. Let's just get the fuck out of here. This party is whack, anyways."

"No shit, I didn't want to come here in the first place. It was your idea, dick."

A few months later, I learned that Jake and some fraternity brothers jumped a Middle Eastern student on campus. I doubted they had the faintest clue about his nationality, not that it mattered. The kid looked different—brown. As he walked across campus, alone at night with just his book bag, they beat the hell out of him and hospitalized the poor kid.

After college, Jake enlisted in the Marines and went to Iraq and Afghanistan. Sure enough, on the night of Alex's engagement party, he had just gotten home from his second tour. Just in time for us to hang out again.

Carl showed up at Alex's with a bottle of Hennessy. He was trying to be thoughtful and commemorate the occasion, so he got something nice, I supposed. But only bottle. I eyeballed the single fifth, lamenting Carl's decision to go with quality over quantity. Alan was on his way, and I thought about calling him to tell him to bring some more alcohol. But I resisted the urge. I didn't want to sound desperate. Plus, I needed to keep myself in check for the night. A slower start would be a strategic one.

Nonetheless, I pretended to go get a snack so I could instead take inventory and see if they had more booze in the kitchen. Plenty of beers. I would have rather had another bottle of whiskey, but we were okay. I took a couple of beers to the bathroom before Alan got there, and I put them down quickly. I rationalized that I should get a little head start just in case I didn't get my share of the sole bottle of Hennessy that would get split four ways. I brought out the rest of the beer for everyone after quickly eating something so they couldn't smell the beer already on my breath.

We drank the whole bottle, along with several beers apiece, while we played a game Alex and I made up called Choose Your Own Adventure. It was a simple game. The captain got to make rules, and the rules had to involve drinking. Then just switch captains and lather, rinse, repeat. My favorite decree as captain was a scavenger hunt. Everyone got a list. Whoever brings the random crap back first wins. Carl's footspeed served him well. Winner. Alex still had a remote control and a stapler to round up. Two drinks for Alex. Alan only brought back a spatula and a basketball, and not much else. Dead last. Five for Alan.

I got a bit more alcohol in me while they rounded up the various household trinkets I'd assigned. *I haven't hit ten yet, have I? No way.*

Probably a lie. I'd also convinced myself I wouldn't drink much more after we left. Another lie.

Before we left, Alex said I needed a better shirt for the bar we were going to. I had on a rag of a t-shirt I'd gotten at a punk rock concert. I liked to wear it at the boxing gym. "Come on, this shirt is fantastic!" I feigned protest.

"Shut up, Dave. You know this is my engagement party, right? Put this on. They won't let you in without it," he said as he pressed a plaid, collared button-down into my chest.

"What? Come on, man. Where did you even get this?"

"It's nice. Banana Republic."

"Fine, if you say so. I think my t-shirt is okay, though."

"It doesn't have fucking sleeves! Just get the shirt on and let's go."

"Fine, I'll wear it," I said as I reluctantly threw it on. Alex weighed about forty pounds more than me. I looked ridiculous in his shirt, like a kid wearing his dad's stuff. I was pretty drunk—we all were—but I was still in control, I thought. I told myself I wasn't going to drink much more. And, more importantly, that I wouldn't lose my head when I saw Jake.

And then, faster than I could keep track, *pretty drunk* quickly turned into *wasted*. I had drunk too much. Too quickly. Faster than the alcohol could mix with my blood. I had maneuvered to make sure I didn't get less than my share of Hennessey, but in the process, I probably got much more. And I wasn't sure how many beers. I let myself lose count so I didn't have to tell myself the truth about how many I'd had.

By the time we left for the bars, everything had started melting around me. Alex, Carl, and Alan had become blurry, hazy figures. The streets we walked down had turned shadowy and obscured. And my demeanor… it had grown irritable, angry, or worse. Moments before, I was in control. But suddenly I was careening chaotically towards a collision with Jake, wherever he was. And, as always, the animal would be lurking, waiting. This was its plan all along.

V

The holiday lights up and down the street are screaming. Dizzy. Drifting.

Walk in a straight fucking line, man.

How long have I been alone? Where are Alex and Alan and Carl? Why did they leave me? What did I do? Motherfuckers. I wish I could rewind and start tonight over again.

Text Annie. Maybe she'll come out. Maybe she can rescue me before the animal takes over.

Any chance you want to come? Maybe we can just hang out for a bit and go home early?

The dots. But no response. Go figure. She doesn't want to see me. Not after last night. I wish I was just home with her. Sober. Clean. I'm losing her. I'm fucking losing her. I can feel it in my chest. I need a touch from her. A hand on my shoulder. Just a light squeeze. But I don't deserve to be with her right now. I don't deserve her at all.

Fuck it. Time for another drink. Stop at a different bar before the party.

I don't know which bar I'm in or how long I've been here. It's crowded. People bumping into me. My friends probably aren't even looking for me anymore. Everyone is going to leave me. Annie. Friends. Fucking everyone. I am so alone. And so angry. Fists clenching tighter and tighter.

Powerful hands on each of my arms are ripping me off my feet. The bouncers are throwing me back to the street. Spitting me out of this place. What did I do? I can't even remember. I'm alone, and they're both fucking big. Fuck this. I need to get to the party anyway.

This place is upscale. Good thing I took Alex's Banana Republic shirt. Everyone is here. Alex and his fiancé. Their friends from high school and college. Families that flew in from wherever. Pleasantries and congratulations and toasts. Blah fucking blah. I'm an outcast. The dregs of this whole fucking party. Why am I even here?

Carl and Alan and Alex. "Dude, sorry, man, we were walking and looked back, and you were just gone…"

Fuck you guys, you ditched me. I don't hear them anymore. Jake's here, I can feel it. My skin is—hotter. My ears, ringing. I hate him so much I can literally fucking hear it. Screeching. Louder and louder.

I see him. Back of the bar. Waiting for a drink, alone.

Pushing my way through the crowd. Inches from him. He looks bigger than before. Stronger.

Say whatever you can think of to make him want to fight you.

I can't even hear myself. I'm fucking ready.

His hand is around my neck. I didn't see it. So fast. Can't pry him loose. Strong motherfucker. I can't breathe. He's an inch away from my face.

"Don't you ever fucking talk about the war."

He's leaving. No, fight me. "Don't walk away!"

Outside now. Street corner looking in each direction. Don't see him. His friend approaching me. This fucking dipshit.

"Fuck you, man!" *He's right in my face.* "What the fuck is your problem?"

The animal in me doesn't care who we fight. "Come on, take a swing at me. I dare you."

He's winding up. But his feet. Bad balance. Too drunk. Or doesn't know how to throw a punch. Take a quick step back. He fell over.

I will hurt you now. Wide stance, feet planted, right hand pulled back and ready.

But—now I'm on the ground instead. Big, heavy bodies on top of me. More of his friends? Can't get up, they're too strong. I can't even move my arms. Who are you? My wrists are twisted and pulled behind me. It's not Jake's friends. Cold metal handcuffs cinching my wrists tight. Police. Fucking hell, not again.

People all around me. Guests from the party, Alex's future in-laws, and random strangers. All watching me scratch and claw at the sidewalk. I can barely breathe. Too much weight on me. Wheezing. Pathetic. I see my friends' faces. Their eyes. What is that? Anger toward me. Sadness for me. Both. I can't look at them.

What the fuck have you done, Dave?

But I can't stop. What difference does it make? I've already fucked everything up. Wrenching my hands apart and let the metal dig into my wrists. More pain. Bring it. Trying to get up from the twisted pile I'm in. But their big knees are planted on my back. Roll to my side, out of under them. I'm running. Five, maybe ten feet. But they're on top of me again.

"Stay down! Do not fucking move!"

Head is firmly crammed into the cement this time. I can't fight anymore. Can't even move. My body is giving in. Getting stuffed into the backseat of the squad car. A bad dog in its cage. I'll be parked back here for a while. Until they break the crowd up. On display through the windows until then. Blue and red flashing lights hitting my face. It's time to hang my head. The animal got its fucking way again. He's satisfied, for now. Leaving me alone with overwhelming fucking shame. I'm scum, scraped off the fucking street. Why couldn't I get out of my own way for just tonight?

There's Alex. I want to tell you I'm sorry. I didn't mean for this to happen. I ruined your special night. You should only have one best man, after all.

I don't deserve a friend like him. Or a partner like Annie. But maybe when she hears about tonight, I won't.

I think I'll understand if you leave me after this.

VI

Stupid questions from the nurse at the station. Telling her whatever can get me lying down fastest. But she's taking forever. While I'm still drunk enough to pass out and make everything—Jake, the police station, Alex's fucking shirt—all just vanish for a few hours. But I'm seeing everything I've done. Drinking too much Hennessy. Getting bounced out of some bar before the party. Jake, in the back, waiting for his drink...

Finally done with the fucking questions. Just fingerprints left. Each finger leaving a mark in their logs. Mine are already buried in one of these books somewhere in here, from the last time I spent the night. Thoughts are racing faster and faster the longer I sit here. Maybe tonight someone cuts me open with something sharp in the cell, and all this pain and shame and guilt can go away. Forever.

It's starting to feel like panic. Or rage boiling over. I want to explode again. Like earlier. Like at the bar with Jake and his fucking friend. I never got to land that punch. I wish I had. I can feel everyone's eyes on me. Not just the people here. The people at the party, friends at dinner parties, and, of course, Annie at home.

You're a fucking virus infecting people, Dave.

In the cell, finally. But it took too long. I can't sleep now. I'll be up all night with these racing thoughts clawing inside my head, trying to get out. The animal is back. He wants to find a target. Someone is going to suffer with me. I want tonight to get worse for me but for someone else, too. Provoke me, anyone.

These three assholes. Right on cue. Tattoos on their arms and necks. Maybe early twenties. They're laughing. Loud. Rowdy.

You want everyone to think you're tough. That you'll be in charge in here until tomorrow morning. That we're stuck in here with you. We'll see about that. You don't know it yet, but you're stuck in here with me, too.

They're fucking with this kid in a striped rugby shirt and khaki pants. Some crap from a J. Crew men's catalog. A DUI arrest. You look too scared, that's why they are fucking with you.

"Move, bro, you're in my seat."

Don't do it. Don't move over. No, you fucking pussy.

"Gotta move again, bro, now you're in *my* seat."

Humiliating him. You fucking hyenas.

"Leave him the fuck alone." *This is a bad idea—three of them and one of me. Too late, though, fuck it.* "Come move me instead, motherfuckers." *Keep looking calm. Barely lifting my head up from Alex's rolled-up shirt.* "Come try it. See what happens." *No plan for when they come over here, but I don't care.*

One is saying something back. Cut him off. "Don't talk back to me, motherfucker. Just stop fucking with that kid." *Adrenaline snapping me to my feet. They're scowling me but not moving yet. Still deciding if I'm too crazy or too fucked up to bother with.*

Keep at it. Make them back down. "What do you want to do, motherfuckers?" *These guys are probably going to fuck me up. But my eyes are burning. Fists are ready. Fingernails digging into my palms. I* want someone to jump. I can't wait. They're talking shit and barking back at me. But they're not coming. "That's right, that's what I thought, you scared motherfuckers."

Laying back down. Eyes closed. My hands between the back of my head and Alex's shirt. They're wondering how confident I really am. If I'm bluffing. A minute or two, now. I guess they're done. I wanted a fight, even though I know I'd lose. But this is satisfying, too. A little wave of relaxation. Maybe I'll fall asleep after all. It would be nice to pass out until I get let out of—

Can't see. Only black. Can't move. Not quite knocked out. But frozen. I didn't see his fist, but I heard it crack me in the face. Warm blood pooling in my eye socket and running down my cheek to the cement. Hands and feet are thundering down on me. I can't feel them. Only my head.

Cover your face. Get onto your hands and knees. Now plant your feet and spring up like a fucking animal. Launching my own punches in all directions. There's still too much blood in my eyes. Connecting some. Missing, too.

One grabs me from behind. Throw this dude off me.

Throwing another punch. And another. But I only see two of them now. Where's the third guy?

My neck. Tattooed forearm is lodged under my jaw and around my throat. Not enough air. I'm leaning backward. Less and less air. Can't see. Fuck I will pass out soon. My heels are propping me up, so I can still kick. Got one right in the balls.

"Fuck you! Fuck all of you!" *Enough air to whisper it. Not gonna stop fighting back. You'll have to choke me out.*

Guards. Ripping us apart. They're strong.

"Everybody back the fuck up!"

A lot of blood on the ground between us. Mine, I think. The split skin over or under my eye is pumping it out fast. On my clothes. My face. It's fucking repulsive in here. Animals. All of us.

"You!"

"Me?"

"Yes, you! Let's go!"

"But they—"

"Shut the fuck up!"

Dragged to a little cell across the hall by myself. I can still see these three motherfuckers. And they can still see me. Ha, perfect. Gang signs with their hands. Shouting whatever the fuck they're shouting. Smile back.

A couple of wrapped gauze squares thrown through the bars into my cell. Not at all enough. I love it. The animal loves it. I don't want to be cleaned up by staff. Don't want to be tended to by a nurse. If there is still even one here. Putting on the gauze myself. Dirty fucking hands. It's already soaked through. Fuck it, it'll stop bleeding sooner or later. Until then, the blood is painting a story on my face.

I'm kind of relaxed after all that. Maybe I can get a bit of sleep.

VII

What time is it? The cell gate's opening. It feels early, but there's no clock down here and no windows. It looks the same as when I fell asleep. No sunlight coming in or out, just fluorescent tubes. Most flickering or burned out.

A fast release this time. I know the routine. Yellow paper bag with my wallet, keys, phone, and belt. Two gates with enough space between them for a person and a guard. One opens, we go in. Then it closes before the second one opens. Like an airlock from a space movie, keeping whatever is on one side from infecting the other.

I see windows at the top of the stairs. The sun is up. Just barely. Shit. The glare is burning my eyes. I'm like some kind of fucking night creature, afraid of the sun. The Sunday morning street is so empty.

"Thank you, officer." Ha, he didn't even look at me.

That bus stop has a clock. Seven a.m. That was a couple hours of sleep at most. Where should I go right now? Can't go home. I can't see Annie like this, with a face that's swollen and cut and clothes that are blood-soaked rags. She's hopefully asleep. Peaceful. Beautiful. She probably doesn't know I got arrested yet. Delay the inevitable for as long as I can.

My hands are disgusting. Dirty. Grimy. Bloody. My face... reflection in a car window. I don't want to look at it, but I should. Dried blood all over. Looks like fucking face paint.

Just remembered, we set up a football game for this morning. It's at ten. I'll run to Alex's parents' house and wake him up. It's at least five miles, I haven't slept, and I just fought three guys in a cell. I could take a cab. But I'd rather run. I'm not stopping until something makes me.

Is it early enough that someone might still be out drunk driving? Maybe I'll run on the street instead of the sidewalk. Maybe that drunk driver won't see me. Maybe I won't see him either. And then maybe I won't ever have to fix any of this.

Get these legs churning. A little stiff. Alex's collared shirt is still tied around my waist. What a great pillow. He won't want it back, now that I can see how much blood is soaked into it. The shirt is reminding me of everything. The whole fucking night. Jake. Fuck you, Jake. I'm definitely the best man that should be cast aside, but he's still an asshole.

Keep this pace. For the past year, I thought he had two best men in his wedding because he felt guilty getting rid of Jake. But it's me. It's been me all along. Because I'm not reliable. Because maybe on the morning of his wedding, I'll be in some jail instead of handing out programs and showing people to their seats like I'm supposed to. Fuck me. I am so fucking late in realizing the obvious. Run faster. And throw this fucking shirt in the next trash can you see.

It's a steep uphill to their house. I should be tiring. But the energy isn't running out. This feels like the day I was running in Rhode Island. The energy isn't real. It's a hollow, illusory fuel. There's a weird, fuzzy filter over my eyes. Everything looks like static on an old TV. But I can still run.

A couple miles down. Maybe halfway there. No more office towers and big complexes. Now it's houses and little apartment buildings. Families inside. Normal people. I hope they wake up, open their blinds, see me, and quickly draw them shut. Vile and repulsive, they'll think. And they'll be right.

Made it to Alex's parents' house. On my tiptoes. Don't make any noise. Shit—what did my foot just knock over? Coat rack. Dammit—now a box of framed pictures. Even louder.

You are a fucking disaster. You should leave these good people alone.

Almost to the kitchen. Water, juice, anything will—

"Ahh! Oh my goodness!" *Alex's mom's shriek is piercing my ears.* "David, you scared the crap out of us. It's so early. What are…"

I knew this was coming once I got close enough for her to see my face.

"Oh, my—your face! What happened to you?"

"I'm fine, don't worry."

"Are you okay? Come here, let me see that!"

She's panicking. Just sound calm. "Totally fine. It looks worse than it is. There's a lot of blood vessels in the face, that's why boxers have all that goopy stuff in their corners." *What? Blood vessels? Boxers? Just stop talking, you idiot.*

There's Alex's dad. "You need to get stitched up! Let's take you to the hospital."

"I just need some water. And some coffee. If you've got it?"

"Come here. Let me at least get this cleaned so it doesn't get infected."

"What happened to you?"

Can't look his dad in the eye. "I just had a bit of a rough night. And sorry for coming in like this. I just wasn't sure where to go."

Alex's footsteps on the stairs. Staring at me from the edge of the kitchen. Looking at me like I'm a thing, not like I'm me.

I look at him. "You ready for the game?"

"Dave... come on. You shouldn't play. Go to the hospital and get stitches. Or at least go home and go to sleep."

"We're going."

"Fine. If you get hurt, though, it's not my fault."

"Fair enough!"

Hurt? I'm already hurt. Everywhere. I don't care. I would rather go play football and get another black eye than go home right now. As far as Annie knows, everything is okay, and I just spent the night here. Not in jail again. I'm not ready for her to see me and then probably leave me. That'll have to wait a few hours.

Silence in the car. Not sure what to say. He's pissed. He should be. I fucked everything up. I should apologize but I don't know how to say it. He doesn't look like he wants to hear anything from me.

Everyone is already on the field. Expressions change as I get closer.

"Let's play!"

No one is arguing with me. They're just staring at me like a car crash. Maybe I should explain. Fuck it. Whatever you all think, I don't care.

My knees. Back. Neck. The numbness from the alcohol has worn off. I feel raw. I'm almost ready to cave in. Swirls of bright light. I'm dizzy.

"Dave, you're done, man, just go take a break."

"No, man, I'm good." *I can see them huddling together and looking in my direction, trying to figure out what to do with me.*

"Okay, whatever. Dave, go deep, fly route." *Trying to put me out of my misery. Well played.*

Running fast, but my feet are banging into each other. Everything is spinning. But the ball should be here soon. Hands out. It bounces off one, then the other. My legs are about to give out.

I'm limp as I crash. Floating for a moment. Rock bottom is only inches away. Dirt and grass, getting into the cuts on my eye and mouth. Past the endzone, in a heap. But it's finally still and quiet. And there's silence in my head. I'm too exhausted even for my thoughts to race. It's almost peaceful...

"Dude, wake up. It's time to go."

Tugging on the back of my t-shirt. Face down in the dirt. They played the rest of the game without me. More tugging. But I don't want to move. The aches in my body—getting up will hurt. And the screaming voice in my head. I don't even want to open my eyes. Scared to.

Things are coming into focus. The blurry brown and green is turning into dirt and blades of grass. And now the night is rushing back. The drinking games. Scavenger hunt. Too much Hennessy. Crowds of people. The grip of the two big bouncers. Hating Jake. Finding him. Then saying something. His hand around my throat. Outside on the street, tackled and cuffed by police. That sad J. Crew kid. Fighting off the three hyenas. And the animal right beside me all night. Snarling and gnashing its teeth.

But what did I say to Jake? It's the one thing that won't replay. I remember his face after I said it. His hand around my neck. Fingers digging in, cutting off the air. My hands, trying to pry his off. Running outside after him. His friend trying to fight me. Falling down. But what the hell did I say to him in the first—

Oh, no.

How could I?

"I wish you'd gotten shot in the desert."

And now it won't stop playing, over and over and over. Fuck you, Dave.

Part Eleven

Chapter 1 - The Quail

When I was a kid, my parents took us to their friend's house in the country every summer for a weekend or two. It was a family of hunters, with a basement full of rifles, ammunition, and homemade venison jerky hanging up to dry. The kids, who were a few years older than me, taught me how to shoot with the old .22 caliber rifle they'd learned on. Using paper targets pinned to bales of hay, I quickly became an excellent shot.

One year, they invited me to come along on an afternoon hunting trip. I didn't really want to go—I'd never shot something that was alive—but I didn't say no. I watched them take down a half dozen birds, rabbits, and other unlucky creatures. I concealed a poignant, sharp pain in my chest every time another bouncy, skittering animal turned into a limp carcass. I couldn't get back to the house fast enough. But as much as I hoped they'd let me remain a spectator, I knew at any moment they'd shove a rifle into my chest, delighted to usher me vicariously through this rite of passage.

"Go for it, city kid! Snag your first kill!" someone said, while a flurry of fingers pointed at a fat quail perched atop the trunk of a fallen tree. "That's an easy shot!"

I gripped the rifle dangling right in front of my hands. It *was* an easy shot, which made it all the worse. It meant I would have to choose whether or not it was going to die. My chest burned as I watched the quail for a moment, hoping secretly it would flap its useless, puny wings and amble away before I could get it into my sights. But it just sat there, chubby and indifferent.

I raised the rifle and slid the butt into the nook of my shoulder. It was the same gun I'd used to sink hundreds of rounds through hay bales in their pasture. I knew how the weight was distributed. I knew how the tired, grainy finish of the wood felt in my fingers. I knew it fired just a tick to the right of the crosshairs. I knew how much pressure it took to engage its spritely hair trigger. And, finally, I knew I'd never miss this fat, meandering quail. Unless I wanted to, that is.

"You got this, David. Go on and get you one!" someone else said.

I pretended to true my aim a bit longer, just to give the oblivious bird one more chance to fly away. But it didn't—it made me decide. I had its breast lined up perfectly in the sights, a touch to the left, exactly where that old .22 wanted it. But on an exhale, I carefully nudged the rifle. Just a degree or two. Not perceptible to my hosts, but enough to miss. I pulled the trigger. A commotion of wood chips and dry leaves. The chubby bird flew away.

"Aww, crap," I lamented. "Next time." There'd be no next time, though. I'd make sure that was both my first and last hunting trip.

That was me—a sensitive kid. Not wanting to hurt things. Even birds, let alone myself or other people. But the afternoon of the quail and the old .22 with the spritely trigger was long ago.

I got home Sunday night, and I took about three times my dosage of antidepressants and mood stabilizers to try to slow down the obsessive thoughts about my own death. I had to talk to Annie. *I'm sure she's heard. Or, if she hasn't, she'll see my fucking face.*

"Hi, babe," I whispered as I walked into the living room.

"Hi." The look on her face—I hadn't seen it before. We'd had dozens of conversations after I'd embarrassed her and plenty more after I'd gotten into real trouble and frightened her. But I knew this was different.

"Are you okay?"

"No, not really," I quickly acknowledged.

"I'm sorry."

"Are you done with me?"

"I'm not going to give up on helping you. But I don't think I do this anymore. I can't watch from up close."

It landed with a thud. *I don't think I can do this anymore.* Too much for my fragile, crippled mind. I didn't have a response. She didn't deserve some false promise that I couldn't back up. I knew she wouldn't accept it, either. I just let my head fall into my hands and started crying instead. She came over and put her hand on my back, waiting. Between the despair and the surge of antidepressants, I passed out.

I knew I'd wake up in the middle of a panic. I could feel it brewing. I could always tell when I was on the verge of another episode, and there was nothing I could do to stave it off. No more than I could change the weather and wish away a storm. So I let myself rest while I had the chance. Of all things, before work the next day, I had an appointment with Dr. Ewing. I didn't feel comfortable with him, but it didn't matter. Maybe he could do something to slow down this freefall.

||

Eyes wide open. Can't move. Trapped. Feels like weight on top of my body. The same feeling from the day I was committed. It's stirring in my head, gathering speed. I have to get up. Can't just lie here wishing this wasn't real. Get up... Get up!

Have to get to the doctor. Running late. No shower. Mouthwash. Water on my face. I can hardly recognize myself in the mirror. Who in the fuck are you, man?

Annie's beautiful face, still sleeping. Don't wake her. Maybe the last time I'll ever see her lying in this bed. I destroyed us. How many fucking warnings did she give me? How many chances? All the patience I could have ever asked for. But I still fucked this up. Because I can't stop. Too scared.

Appointment is in thirty minutes. No time to park. Fuck it. Just get a parking ticket. I can't miss it. I need a refill on the prescriptions. I think I'd be dead by now without them. But I don't even let them work. They're fucking diluted with whiskey and shit.

I need more than a refill. I need to talk. Need help. I'm drowning. I don't remember what normal feels like. I'm always depressed, manic, drunk, or angry. Tell him what happened. Maybe he'll point me in a direction, any direction. Or grab me and lock me up like Phil did in Rhode Island that day I tried to fucking die. I'm panicking. Fuck. Try to relax. Breathe.

The line's not moving at all. The woman in front of me. Fuck. Small talk with the receptionist. Please just hurry, lady, I can't miss this appointment. Annie's words are tearing through my head. Over and over and over.

"I can help you over here!"

Another receptionist. About fucking time.

She smiles and says, "Good morning."

I can't speak. Not with this huge lump in my throat. If I speak, I'll burst into tears. Trying to smile back.

Ten minutes late. Should be okay. But I wish I had the whole thirty minutes. I need him to do something. Send me somewhere. Lock me up in a room and just not let me hurt myself anymore. Prescribe something that makes me allergic to booze. If there were such a thing.

Why hasn't he called me in yet? He usually buzzes me in by now. The receptionist is supposed to push a button or something. Maybe she forgot? Calm down. It's been thirty fucking seconds. Deep breath.

Still nothing. He can't be running late. He's too uptight to be late. The receptionist must not have pinged him. I'm gonna knock. What the fuck else am I supposed to do?

"Doctor Ewing?"

Nothing? Is he not even here? It didn't even matter that I was late, after all. But this isn't the day for him to miss the appointment. Because I'm going to be out of pills. Because I'm scared. Because I don't know what I'm going to do next.

A little louder. "Doctor Ewing?" Still nothing. I need your help. I'll head back to the receptionist and see if—

The door. Just a sliver of his face showing, like he's hiding from me. "David, you'll need to reschedule for another date."

What? No, please. "But it's only nine-fifteen, I have until nine-thirty. I'll just do a short appointment."

"You know I don't see patients late. We've discussed this before, David. You can reschedule downstairs or call in."

"What do you mean? How can you turn me away right now? Look at me! I need help!" *Pressing my finger into the black and blue flesh underneath my eye. It hurts. Press harder. And harder. Searing with pain. Tears well up and run down my cheek.* "Do you not fucking understand?"

"Please reschedule."

"But you motherfuckers are always late! How many times have I sat in the fucking waiting room at this fucking hospital waiting for one of you? Now I'm a few minutes late and you're sending me away?"

"Sorry, but you'll have to make another appointment. Now I'm asking you to leave. Goodbye."

Deadbolt.

"Motherfucker!"

Punching the door until skin peels away from my knuckles. Crying. I can't stop. On my knees. Fuck him. I know I don't deserve his help, but I needed it this morning.

My eyes are all emptied out. And inside of me, too. The place deep down. Where all my fucking courage was. Gone. Just like Annie will be.

The abandoned campsite. Watching the knife press down, stretching the skin. Pressing harder, looking for the breaking point...

They're going to call security. I need to leave.

Chapter 3 - Ringing in the New Year

Whatever little resilience still lingered in me had finally given way to fear. Fear of what I would do without a drink. And that fear was costing me a companion. So, I redoubled my commitment to my *other* companion, alcohol. It could never leave me. It couldn't be embarrassed of me. *Until I'm gone, you will always be here for me.*

It was New Year's Day. I was at home, hungover, bleary-eyed. I'd been out all night before, but I wanted to leave again. The apartment, every square inch of it, made me think of Annie and what I'd put her through. She'd been keeping her distance from me. Whenever I opened the door, I wondered if it would be the day I'd find it empty of all her things. Every last shirt, sock, and earring.

I was hanging from a ledge with just one finger. Waiting for someone to just peel it off. My mornings were spent clearing the fog in my head. My days—painful and lonesome. If I wasn't drinking, I wanted to be. If someone didn't want to drink with me, I'd find someone else, maybe, or just drink alone. I wasn't happy when I was drinking. Usually, the animal took hold of me, escalating me to rage. Or, instead, numb indifference.

I wasn't without self-awareness. I knew full well what I'd let myself become. I'd fought back, but I'd lost. I tried with groups, I tried with Paula, and I even tried with Dr. Ewing. I'd tried but given up. I didn't fight with everything in me. And so, defeated, I gave up and gave in, one piece of my life at a time.

I hadn't been hitting the heavy bag at the gym. I hadn't gone running in months. I had put on my running shoes a couple of times and tightened the laces. But all I could do was just sit on the couch with my head in my hands. I bailed on Isaiah. I was supposed to pick him up the prior Sunday morning to help him do some homework and then see a movie. But I'd gotten too wasted and forgot. I went to work just enough to cover my bills. Whatever hopes my mentors at the real estate firm had for me, I was sure they were dashed.

I contemplated death often. Dark invasions of my mind. Thoughts of drinking bottles and bottles and disappearing forever. Of alcohol flowing in and pain flowing out. I thought of a bullet sinking, painlessly, into my head and ending the noise. I imagined my funeral, being an invisible guest, and observing the crowd's unspoken ambivalence.

With Annie, these imaginations had subsided. The goodness in her, it tamped down those burning, desperate impulses. But I knew leaving was the best thing for her. *It will be easier for us both if I just submit and let the big waves swallow me.*

It was a quiet afternoon in the city on New Year's Day. The streets were tired from the raucousness of the night before. I had plans to meet an old friend from Dartmouth, Betsy, who was in town for the holidays. She hadn't seen me in years. If she had, she'd have known to find someone else to meet up with.

It was only the afternoon, but I wasn't going to wait for her to start drinking. I scrolled through my phone's contacts list, top to bottom. I tried my good friends—those that I still had. But I also tried loose acquaintances—near-strangers I'd eagerly swapped phone numbers with. But no one called me back. *Fuck you. I don't need anyone.*

Eventually I got a response from a college classmate named Jesse. He said he would meet me at the Final Stop, a bar we all knew. I knew it was pity. My pride might have previously stopped me from begging people to hang out with me. But not anymore. I cared less about what anyone thought *of* me. It mattered more simply whether they were drinking *with* me.

Whenever I hung out with Jesse, I felt like he was on the verge of saying something. It was the way he looked at me—his head tilted up, his eyes narrow, like he was studying me, forming his words. *It's better that you don't say what you're thinking. Don't make me choose. It won't be you.*

I was drinking my first glass of whiskey when they arrived. Jesse got himself a beer. Even though he was drinking with me, it seemed that his sips were measured and reluctant.

"Dave, how are you, man?" he asked, once there was no one in earshot. The inflection made it sound like something other than a question. He put his big paw on my shoulder and squeezed.

You already know the answer. Why ask? I'm fucking terrible, man. "Great! New Year's Day." I didn't look him in the eye when I spat out that unconvincing lie.

"We're worried, man."

Well, shit. "Uh, I mean, it's been a bit of a rough stretch lately, I guess."

A new text. *Saved by the bell.*

"Oh, hey, James is on his way over!"

Soon, the three of us were all talking and drinking whiskey or beer. Jesse abandoned the topic of my well-being and the three of us instead talked NBA hoops and occasionally raised a new, full glass to the New Year. I wished I could somehow press pause at that moment and live in that hollow still-frame. But as the late afternoon rolled into the evening, and the bar began to fill up, Jesse headed home.

"James! Don't leave yet! I'm meeting Betsy. Remember her? You should come!" I threw my hands up in the air, clumsily splashing a little whiskey on the way.

"I don't think so, man. I'm beat," he said.

"Okay, well let's just hang out here a bit longer, alright?" *I don't want to be alone right now, please.*

We played a game of darts and had another drink. I knew he was placating me, squeezing beers into his already uneasy stomach. I appreciated the companionship. It staved off solitude for a bit longer.

"Okay, I really gotta turn in. I'm wiped," he finally conceded.

"I know. It's okay. Thanks for staying."

"Are you gonna be okay? Maybe you should just head home yourself."

"I'm fine. I mean—no, I'm not doing great. But I can't go home."

"Yes, you can. I'll take you there myself."

"I can't. I just can't be there right now," I admitted. "It's just too late, I think."

"Too late for what? I don't like the way you're sounding. I'm worried about you. Everyone is."

"I don't know. But, I love you, brother. Happy New Year," I said, before we pulled each other in for a hug.

I spent another hour at the bar drinking by myself. But I wasn't really any more alone than before. I still had my truest companion of all. And now it was just the two of us. The heavy glass moved as if a part of my hand, while the amber liquid was part of my blood. The drink and I were engrossed in each other, absolutely.

I melted away for a few more rounds, before leaving my car and hopping in a cab to a bar called the North Star to meet Betsy. I was completely awash in alcohol. Hard, fast drinking. The kind not meant to dampen pain, but to numb it entirely.

IV

"Huh?" *I think the cab driver said something to me.*

"I said, we're here. Twelve, even. Are you okay? You look like you're going to pass out, man."

"Here's twenty. And mind your own business."

"Just trying to help, asshole."

Overwhelming here. Disoriented. Close to blacking out. Cabbie was right. Music, people, lights—all moving too fast. Go get another shot. And a Red Bull while you're at it. Wake the fuck up.

Betsy. "Hey!"

She doesn't know me anymore. She thinks I'm normal.

"Hi, guys! Happy New Year!"

Her boyfriend, whatever his name is. "Yes! Happy fucking New Year! Dave, how have you been?"

He's talking to me like we're best buds. Feels good.

"Fucking fantastic! Been forever, huh? Let me get us all some shots." *I barely remember you. But you can be my best friend tonight if you can keep up.*

Shots for everyone. An extra for me. Quickly, before they see. Her boyfriend is too close to my face. I can smell his breath. Can't quite hear him, but he's laughing. I'll laugh, too. Annie, my friends, my boss, none of them are here. I'm anonymous. And it's only midnight. I won't stop. Tonight, I want to sink into a sea of alcohol and find out how deep it goes.

Another hour. Shots and another round of beers. Don't know what time it is. It's so crowded. Other bodies are keeping me from falling down.

Another hour. Or more. I can't see clearly. Can't quite think. But I'm still standing. So, I can still drink.

Shots again. Jamison.

Blaring strobe lights. Betsy's favorite song.

Stepping outside. Cold air, a cigarette.

But things are disappearing.

And now... nothing.

V

Fuck. The sun. My eyes. It's dawn. I'm on my couch. I was at the North Star and then—now I'm here. What the fuck was in between I don't know. My heart's pounding. Usually there is something. An image or two. But there's absolutely fucking nothing. I keep getting stuck on that last fucking shot of Jamison and a cigarette. No memories after that. I am fucking scared.

Everything hurts. Head, arms, legs. Hand is wrapped in bandages. And is this blood on my clothes? Don't want to but need to look in the mirror. Blood, bruises, and a black eye. Under these bandages? Fuck —it looks like a maze of little cuts and shards of glass.

The bruises—fists and feet or elbow and knees. What else could they be? But how the fuck could I not remember this? If I can't remember getting beat up, what else is missing?

Phone. No texts, but called Will at three. Where the hell was I at fucking three? Nothing is even open after two. And how did I even get back here? No receipts in my pocket or wallet from a cab. Bus doesn't run that late. Credit card charges? This slow fucking computer... hurry the fuck up. No charges for taxis so maybe Betsy sent me home and paid. But then I would have gotten home sooner. What the fuck were you doing, man? I don't know... I don't know... I do not fucking know!

I have to go get my car from—fuck me. Sticky, dried blood all over my keys. From my own hand, right? Okay, I need to relax so I can fucking think. But nothing makes sense. I didn't take a cab or bus. I couldn't have walked. That's five fucking miles...

You didn't drive home, did you?

So many bullshit promises that I wouldn't do it again. All of them, broken. But I've never done it without remembering anything. An image. Shiny tiles in the Broadway Tunnel. The feeling when I floor it on the bridge. But this—this vacuum—is something new. No, I couldn't have. I'd remember something. My car must still be way across town. But I need to check.

It's cold out. Jog. No sign of it on Twenty-Eighth Street. Twenty-Ninth... nothing. So much fog. I can only see three or four cars in front of me. Two blocks and I'm already dizzy, fucking hell. It's not hard to park on the weekends. I wouldn't have had to go any farther. Okay, breathe. Almost there. Just check a few more cars and then I'll be able to calm the fuck—

Oh, no. How could you? Are you trying to get someone killed? You deserve to die yourself, you motherfucker. A deep burning in my chest. I want to claw it out. Okay, slow down, look around. I don't see any dents so no wreck. And I'm not in jail, so I didn't get pulled over. Maybe something inside will help me remember.

Oh, my God, fuck. More blood. All over the handle and all over the door. Maybe this is a dream. Please let me wake from this. No. This is real. The mist, the wet sidewalk—it's all real. This isn't a nightmare. This is just—this is you.

Heart is racing scary fast. Whose fucking blood is this? Please be mine. Pretty fucking please, God, be mine. More on the seats and the steering wheel. On the seatbelt and the buttons. Maybe it's all from my hand, but I don't think—there's so much. I don't know. It doesn't make sense. I'm losing it.

What if I hit someone? Shit, what if someone is watching right now? Get the fuck inside, man.

This slow, old Mac. Hurry up, fuck. Nothing on the SF Chronicle website. Nothing anywhere on the SFPD site either. Paranoid? I don't think so. But I don't fucking know. Everything is aching. I need to lie down. Hard to keep my eyes shut. Too fucking panicky. But just keep them shut until you pass out. It's not working. Too much... chaos.

A shower. Wash this off me. The blood. The cold sweat. The night that's stuck to me. Water as hot as I can stand. I want to melt the outer layer of me away and wash it down the drain. Can't stand up.

Was I asleep? The water's cold. I'm in a ball.

I don't want to keep going. Death is in front of me. One way or another. I feel myself closing in on it. Faster and faster. I'm about to crash. Is that going to be the story of me? Am I going to let myself die? Or do I have any fight left? Any fucking courage at all? I don't know. But it's now or never. That's for goddamn sure.

Annie's voice. I need to hear it. She's the only one. The only one that can help me find that courage if it's even still there.

Please pick up.

She's staring at it, somewhere. Deciding to let it go to voicemail or not.

"Are you okay?"

"No. I'm not at all okay."

"Are you hurt? Is someone hurt?"

"I don't know, honestly. I can't remember anything. There was blood on me when I woke up, and—"

"Jesus, babe. What the fuck happened? You're scaring me."

"It doesn't matter anymore. It doesn't matter because it stops now. I want to stop for you. Just give me a chance. I swear I can do it."

"David, you can't stop for me. You need to do it for yourself. Whether I'm with you or not." *I think she's crying.*

"I know. But with you, I think I *can* do it for myself. For both of us."

"I can't keep waiting. It's so hard to watch. I just can't…"

"I can do it. I can stop. Now. I don't know how yet, but I'll do it. I'll fight harder than I ever have fought before. I love you so much, please don't leave just yet. Just—not yet. I can do this. I will do this."

There's light shining through. By a thread but hanging on. It won't be for nothing. Because if I don't change, she's gone. Then, probably, so am I. I'm not ready to give up. I'm not ready to die.

I have to fight.

Chapter 6 - Bcc:

I usually spent Monday mornings wringing my conscience dry of whatever I did while binging all weekend. Trying to scrub myself clean, just to start the cycle all over again. But not this time. Something was different. The imminence of my danger to others, including Annies, had never been clearer. What if I had killed someone else? "There's been an accident." What if someone had to hear those ominous words, because of me? What if a mother or father or husband or wife had to identify a body after I destroyed a life while driving drunk and blind across the crowded city? This reality had been in plain sight, of course, but my mind had always found ways to obscure it just enough to let it subsist for another day. And another. I already knew that I needed to change. But never before had I been certain that I *could*.

I hadn't felt hope like this in years. Not since I was eighteen, maybe, leaving for Dartmouth and imagining myself in a circle on the quad, reading Walt Whitman. Before the quick six in Sigma house started a little fire that would smolder, grow, and eventually rage. But that Monday, I saw the truth. I'd become an alcoholic, truly dependent on a substance to numb my pain and mask my illness. *Will that be the story of me? Or will I fight?*

And so, all at once, that Monday morning, I could see everything. I could see myself driving around the city, too drunk to even stand. I could see myself fighting strangers, bouncers, even cops. I could see myself bruised, cut, jailed, beaten. I could see myself terrifying Annie, my friends, my family. Dragging them along that treacherous road with me. Bailing me out of jail. Picking me up from a heap on the sidewalk. Using them to keep me alive. They were like guardian angels. Except they'd never consented to that. *I should be fucking dead or locked away. Everyone will be safer. Unless I put a stop to this, once and for all.*

Wednesday. Three days since I'd had a drink. I went to see Paula. I told her everything—the weekend, the blood, the car, and that it had all finally led me to believe that maybe, just maybe, I could quit. Before that day, Paula had always refrained from telling me that if I ever wanted to be healthy, I would simply have to abstain. That there could never be a "relationship" with drinking, only a cold, acrimonious divorce. She probably knew that until then, I had never been ready to hear it. She was right. But she wasn't seeing the person who would have retreated. She was seeing someone new, someone ready to grit his teeth and prepare to fight.

"I never want to feel this way again. I don't want to hurt anyone. I don't want to lose Annie. I want my life to be more than this."

Paula seized on the spark of courage. "You have to stop drinking, David, or you will not survive."

You will not survive. Her words sent a shiver through me. From my throat to my chest to the pit of my stomach.

"I'm ready," I said, hunched over in my chair, my forehead pressing against my clenched fist. I didn't want to look at her. My face looked like a mess of half-healed bruises and, now, tears.

"Just start with a few more days. Get to Monday. Give yourself that. And I'll see you back here, then."

"Yes, I can do that. I will do that, I mean." I made myself look her in the eye when I said it, steeling my resolve.

"I'll see you very soon, David," she said, "I believe in you."

As I drove over the Bay Bridge to the office, I felt different. The colors around me were changing. The sun was brighter. The water was blue and reflective. Not the gray void I often pictured myself sinking into. I'd thought of stopping before. And I'd tried cutting back or taking breaks. But I'd always surrendered to the physiological addiction, the psychological dependency, and to the absolute and overwhelming fear of life without alcohol. But this was a new day.

When I had tried to just moderate in the past, like the months before my race with Will, I'd always kept my efforts quiet. It was easier to give up on myself in private. I wondered, what would happen if I said it out loud? Would I still retreat? No, I reckoned, I wouldn't allow myself. I'd endure, like I did for my teammates, no matter how much it hurt.

So I started an email, addressed to Annie and my best friends. But that wasn't enough. I wanted to reach far and wide, so I added a few more friends and my family. Still feeling like I was tiptoeing, I piled even more on top of that. Before long, I'd added damn near everyone who was saved in my Gmail contacts. No more privacy. I was going to stand up and scream it out loud. It was the only way. What I wrote was rough, raw, and real. It was as honest as I'd been with myself–or anyone–in years. *Maybe I should call Annie before I send it and see what she thinks.* No. It was time to jump off this cliff.

From: David Shamszad
Subject: [no subject]

Bcc: [undisclosed recipient list]

Friends,

This last Sunday I woke up with blood all over me. I was all cut up and bruised. I can't remember anything that happened Saturday night. Nothing. I didn't know I drove myself home until I found blood inside of the car too. I don't know whose. All of it mine, I hope.

I have a problem. I've been telling myself that I can manage it. Moderate it. Stop after a few drinks. It hasn't worked. Believe me, I've tried. I know now that I have to spend some time without a drop of alcohol in my body. There's not another way. How long it will take, I have no idea. Until I can be sure that I don't need it, I suppose. That could take a long time. That might be forever.

I think I need your help with this. Remember not to offer me a beer. Do things with me at places where there isn't anything to drink. And just know how important this is to me. Maybe my life depends on it. I appreciate you reading this email. It was hard to write, and I'm not sure how I'm going to feel after I hit 'send.'

Love,
David

I was exposed, vulnerable, and open. Doubts swirled. *Maybe I shouldn't have sent that. Maybe I should have watered it down some. Maybe I just freaked everyone out and no one will even want to talk to me again.* The minutes passed very, very slowly. Then the first email came. It was Jesse. He'd wanted to say more on New Year's Day. He could have, but it wouldn't have mattered. I wasn't listening.

I'm proud of you, he wrote. *I have your back, brother. Call anytime you need to talk.*

Then the next one. From my friend who'd hosted the dinner party and given the *look.* I hadn't spoken to him since. I'd been holding a silly, petulant grudge anchored in denial.

We can go to as many movies as you want man, he wrote. *Is* Fast Five *out yet!? Seriously, this is a great thing. Proud of you.*

More and more came in. I was revitalized by the burst of love and support. I didn't know what daunting obstacles stood in front of me or how hard they'd be. But in that moment, the encouragement from my community invigorated me more than I could have ever imagined.

By the end of the workday, I still hadn't heard from Annie. But when I got home late that afternoon, there she sat, waiting in the living room. She stood up and skipped over to me when I walked through the door, before burying me in a deep squeeze. In my ear, she whispered, "I'm here."

"I'm not going to let you down," I said, tears streaming from my eyes.

"I know."

Part Twelve

Chapter 1 - Before the Dawn

I made it to the following Monday and trudged into the second week without alcohol. My body reeled from it—I was chilly, sick, and wrought with headaches. And my mind ached for it—recurring nightmares tormented me. I'd dream I was at a party, a bar, or any place with alcohol on hand. I'd take a few shots. Then a few more. Then end up doing coke in a bathroom, having sex with a stranger, or getting in a fight. When my eyes opened, I'd wake in a dreary limbo, unsure of reality, thinking I'd thrown it all away and relapsed. Guilt lingered with me all day after those dreams. That's how much I feared falling off the wagon. I felt guilty for even dreaming of it.

I was recluse. I didn't have the energy or clarity to talk to anyone or do anything. I hadn't been outside of the apartment except to go to work, which seemed like enough of an undertaking. My friends had reached out, but I didn't want to see them yet. Annie gave me as much attention as she could, day and night. But I didn't want to be a constant burden. I owed her so much more than making her my babysitter or therapist. And I couldn't lean on my friends every night—they had their own shit to do.

After a few weeks, the noisy, physical pain had waned and some of the mental fog had lifted. But it yielded to an omnipresent guilt. Wading through my remorse with a sober head haunted me. My memory became clearer, like an out-of-focus lens on a camera finally locking in on its subject. I could see my friends cleaning me up and wiping vomit or blood from my face and body. I could see my family, wondering if they'd lost their son to the same addiction that plagued my father.

I started with my close friends, apologizing for the embarrassing, sordid, and dangerous situations I'd put them in. I called Alex to apologize, again, for fucking up his engagement party and thank him for still letting me be in his wedding. He said it was okay, that he'd never judged me, and that I was still one of his best friends. I called Will to tell him I was sorry, again, for getting him arrested and thrown in jail. He said not to worry about it, that it'd been two years, and that I'd apologized two hundred times.

"I know, but it just still feels awful. I can see it all so much more clearly now, and I just can't believe I put you through that. It's fucking terrible."

"But it's over. You're better for it. Because it led you here, before it was too late. Just don't give up. I'm here for you, whenever you need."

I also called old acquaintances that weren't my friends anymore—people who had long since written me off. I apologized for things I had done weeks, months, and years prior. Some people told me I need not carry it with me. But some expressed less of a willingness to forgive.

Chelsea, a friend at Dartmouth, had a party when she moved to San Francisco. The next day, I didn't remember anything after the vicodin I popped and the flask of whiskey I finished on the drive over. I'd found out that I'd pushed one of Chelsea's friends after getting into an argument about whose turn it was to play beer pong. I left after she kicked me out, but not before hitting the guy and flipping the table over, showering her patio and several guests with dozens of cups of cheap beer. She wasn't ready to accept an apology.

"Maybe down the road," she said, "but not now."

It was a scar, like many others I'd added over the years. Some had become visible reminders, like the ones I had over one eye and under the other. But most were inside, indelible nonetheless. It would have been easier not to think about what I'd done, but that wasn't me. I made myself stand in the fire and feel it burn.

More than anything or anyone else, I thought of Annie. I could finally see her, as if from above, on all those nights I wasn't there. I could see her scared, wondering—hoping—that I was safe. Asking herself, *How much longer can I do this?*

There's a dark, mucky place a hundred feet below rock bottom. Even as I recklessly tried to claw my way to those suffocating depths, Annie didn't abandon me. Not even for her own well-being. She sat there with me in the pitch black, believing in me still, loaning me her courage when all of mine had diminished. Like a rope thrown to me before I drowned, her belief pulled me out of that muck. Most people wouldn't have stayed, but she did. I thanked her, over and over, every goddamn day. I was overjoyed that a new beginning awaited. But first, I had more work to do. She'd helped me up, but I had to learn to stand on my own.

Chapter 2 - Midnight Basketball

By the time I reached the two-month milestone, I was still fairly secluded. I couldn't yet go back to the places or see the people that triggered deep, relentless impulses to drink. The burning scent of liquor. The loud pop of cold beer bottles opening. The deep, glistening, crimson hue of a glass of wine. They all pulled at me with an unbearable gravity. I worried that if I got too close, my feet might leave the ground.

The pull scared me. *What if this impulse to drink never goes away? Will I turn into a fucking hermit every night? And what if people realize they like things better without me around?* The fear of isolation, of slipping into the shadows of my friends' memories, felt threatening and formidable. But worse yet, looming in the distance, behind that fear of isolation, was the greatest fear of all. *What will I do when I need a drink?* A simple question—yet imminently terrifying.

I'd needed to drink to socialize. I'd needed to drink—a lot—when I saw my family. I'd needed alcohol when I felt mania surging. And I'd needed it when I felt depression taking hold. A drink was a steady promise of certainty amidst the difficult or the unknown. I knew that I had only one way to get out of that cycle. I had to learn to live without alcohol, one day at a time. And then I'd make those days melt into a new life.

But I still couldn't imagine what that life would look like. I didn't know how I could feel better without drinking to numb myself. I didn't know how to spend my time. I didn't know how to be with people. I didn't even know how to be alone. I didn't know how to simply… *be*. But an idea slowly took hold. Maybe instead of just fighting against the inertia of my old ways, I could fight to embrace new ones. Perhaps I could become more and do more with my mind and body. I blindly clung to that idea, letting it propel me from one day to the next.

I got better and better at battling the urge to drink. Each urge I quelled became another arrow in my quiver. I found activities to do to pass time a bit easier. I'd always liked movies as much as anyone, but when

I stopped drinking, I became a buff. Annie came with me to the good ones. I roped other friends into the shitty ones. And for the really bad ones, when no one else wanted to partake, I happily went by my damn self. After the movie, I shared my takes on a Tumblr blog. About a Jake Gyllenhaal movie with a time-machine and a hijacked train, I offered my readers this keen insight: *Best time-travel movie since Ashton Kutcher's* The Butterfly Effect*!* It entertained me, if not my exceedingly small online following.

But the gym is where I put in the most work of relearning how to spend time and feel good doing it. Plus—I'd gotten quite soft. It had been a long, long time since I trained every day for rowing and had any real discipline. The days of a lean, fit, hundred-and-ninety-pound athlete had long disappeared. The waning exercise plus the toxic influx of alcohol nearly every day had left my body weaker than that first day of crew practice. I was soft, slow, and sedentary. And up to two-twenty.

I usually went at night to fill the empty slots. Eventually I went six times a week. Running. Basketball. Weights. Boxing. I did whatever I could get my hands on. I liked to go late on Fridays and Saturdays, using 24 Hour Fitness's robust schedule to give me something to do during the times I usually stayed out drinking. I found a group of regulars that played hoops until one a.m. every Saturday. Maybe they wanted to stay away from bars, like me, I thought. Or maybe they were, also like me, just basketball junkies.

Alex would join me at the gym a few times a week. He was immensely supportive of me when I quit and vowed to do whatever he could to help. And so we leaned into our shared affinity for indulging in tough, nasty workouts. We replaced the days and nights of blacking out together with punishing—though exhilarating—sessions in the weight room, stairs, and, my favorite, the track at Kezar Stadium, original home of the San Francisco 49ers.

Before long, my body became mine again. I celebrated by pushing myself harder. I signed up for more races, usually with Will. They would eventually become an annual tradition that would last years and years. I had feared that our friendship would change when I quit drinking. It was, after all, ultimately how we spent so much of our time together. We did it before every Scrabble match we played, every movie we saw, and every basketball game we watched. I wondered what else we'd do if we couldn't replace it?

But we tore through that fear. We replaced drinking benders with runners' highs. We kept playing Scrabble, though—and scored much, much higher. When I stopped drinking, he also cut back. In the end, all we lost was a shared codependent and destructive habit. The brotherhood we established at nineteen years old—doing hard stuff on the crew team together—formed the true bedrock of our friendship, not the gallons of cheap whiskey we guzzled.

Exercise became nearly compulsory at times, but it was better than the gnarly addictive clutches of alcohol. I became a little edgy if I didn't get a workout in. Sometimes I showed up late to other obligations on account of trying to squeeze a run into impossibly short windows. Exercise had become the most important new routine for me. It all circled back to puking at that first suicides workout and feeling fantastic as my stomach heaved. Or running stadiums the first week of crew practice my Freshman Fall, and feeling overjoyed that I couldn't walk.

Those days out on the water in a boat were when I felt most comfortable in my skin—other than when I drank, of course. So, perhaps, I naturally found refuge in the gym, on the road, or otherwise enmeshed in the connection between my mind and body. Exercise gave me a way to feel strong and good and clean. But the power lay in the routine of it—because it made those feelings available to me every day.

Chapter 3 - Tiki Torches

Without my addiction overshadowing everything else, it was as if Annie and I met for the first time. My love for her had ultimately been competing with love for my vicious drinking habit. I had not earnestly been a part of her life; I had been too selfish for that. I soon realized I didn't know *her* as much as I had known the parts of her I could *use*. I knew she was trusting—which I used to lie. I knew she was forgiving—which I used to evade. I knew she was introverted—which I used to escape. But I didn't know *her*. I didn't know how much she missed her family's old home on a lake in Canada. I didn't know she longed to leave her job and pursue a dream of opening her own business. I didn't even know she wanted to get a dog.

When we went out to dinner, I no longer waited for her to go to the bathroom so I could skip over to the bar for a quick shot. When I looked at her, I no longer looked *through* her. I'd been present, yet imminently absent. We began talking again. Laughing. Discussing the future. Reconciling the past.

"I don't think I'd be here, if not for you."

"Come on."

"No, I mean that. You were my last hope."

"Well, I hope this is just the beginning."

"Oh, you bet your ass."

As the weeks went by, we talked more, walked more, dined more, and danced more. I loved every minute of it. It reminded me of our early days together in Rhode Island, with a thrilling electricity between us and a surety that we were the luckiest people on earth for having found each other.

Perhaps I should have waited, so that she could see my changes would sustain. But my head and my heart were as clear as they were impatient. The toxins had washed away. She was not the crutch I leaned on while I got better. She was the reason why. I knew I wanted to be with her forever and that I'd never love another the same. One Saturday evening in the chilly San Francisco summer, about six months into our new life, I asked her to meet me at the beach. I'd lit up a row of bamboo torches, and I stood waiting with an engagement ring.

"Hey, love."

"Ummm... What is this?"

I got down on one knee. She brought her hands to her face.

"Will you marry me? I want to be with you, and only you, forever."

"Yes, love, I will."

We held each other for minutes on end, closer and closer, erasing every small space between our bodies until the cold air had taken enough of a toll. We then went to dinner on the Embarcadero at a restaurant well outside of our budget.

"You know, the tiki torches were... a bit much," she said with a grin.

She was right. I smelled of lighter fluid and my hands had soot on them that I couldn't scrub all the way off. We were sure the waiters and upscale patrons around us could smell it.

A few months later, we adopted Bodie. Before then, I couldn't have been trusted to care for him. Rescuers had discovered him in the basement of an abandoned home, emaciated and nearly dead. He had fierce separation anxiety and extreme behaviors caused by the trauma he'd endured. I understood why six families gave up on him before us—as I would have understood if my fiance and friends had given up on me. It was the beginning of our family, one of healing, acceptance, and love.

Chapter 4 - A Group of One

At work, I ran on all cylinders for the first time in my adult life. I got to the office at eight a.m. with a clear head, which I'd so rarely afforded myself. Settling into my desk in the morning became fun—*What can I achieve today?*

I had lived with restraints on my hands and feet. No, not lived—survived. Alcohol paralyzed and trapped me just like the handcuffs and jail cells I found my way into. Alcohol restrained my intelligence, ability, and judgment, leaving me unequipped to perform my best or even close to it. And, worse yet, I hadn't truly acknowledged it. Somehow, denial persuaded me that alcohol and an absence of self-care were *not* the reasons my new real estate career had yet to get out of the gates.

But once sober, I became assertive and increasingly confident. I picked up the phone earlier, doubling my volume of calls. Even better, the prospective clients on the other end of the line talked to someone with enthusiasm, drive, and growing competence. I started believing I could expand my territory and venture into bigger and harder transactions.

When an old building hit the market for sale, I approached a client who was in the business of redeveloping older properties. I hadn't brokered a sale transaction this big before—not even close. An earlier version of me would have seen the opportunity but not ventured forward. *This is out of my league. Other guys are more experienced and qualified for this... leave it to them.* But I believed in myself again and knew I could do it if I worked hard enough and . *Why not me? I have to start somewhere, sometime. Why not here and now?*

First, I helped my client determine the costs to restore the building. Then, I pieced together a projection to ascertain the building's potential for profit after considering the cost of the property, the renovations, and expensive interest payments. Once we determined a narrow but viable pathway to reinventing a once-prominent commercial property, I dug in and negotiated a deal for him to buy it. I had to manufacture some courage to write an offer so far below the purchase price and sell our vision, expertise, and commitment to close the deal.

"I know it's low—but my guy can fucking close!" I bellowed during the final call before they ultimately decided to give us the deal.

While he embarked on the construction, I created a marketing plan for the office space and began shopping it to prospective businesses. Before the building was even completed, I'd gotten half of it leased. I'd stayed so busy working on the project that I hadn't entirely stopped to take inventory of what had happened. It was the most significant feat I'd done in the business to that point. More remarkably, it only took the ambition to do something big, the confidence to believe I could do it, and the determination to work it through the finish line. I possessed none of these traits while in the throes of a destructive and debilitating self-medication and addiction.

But I didn't stop long to celebrate. I loved the feeling of success. It felt better than any high, and it reinforced the idea that the change I'd just made in my life paved the way to more of it. Every day, I fought the urge to drink. But the tangible results made it easier, and I could point to them when I needed a reminder. *You just did THAT. What else might be possible?*

I valued and appreciated the opportunity I had to work at the firm, and I wish I'd done more for them during my time there. For several years, they got little from me but my shadow. I felt compelled to stay and show them my potential. But, in my heart, I knew that I needed to start anew. The elevator, the halls, and my desk served as reminders of how I used to feel every morning of every day: sick with nausea or shame —or both.

Maybe that big deal that I'd just completed did it. Maybe it was the wave of confidence that swelled after a few months of not drinking and getting shit done. But a nearly irrational idea occurred to me. *If those guys started a business all those years ago, when they were my age, can't I?* A few weeks later, before I could see the myriad holes in this half-baked plan, I told the firm I planned to leave.

I had a bit of money from the office building deal. Enough to get a small space, a desk, computer, and perhaps half of whatever else I would need to properly start a business. In lieu of a built-out business plan, I had a fucking tornado of enthusiasm and I set out to take my shot. I gave myself a huge incentive to make sure it worked: if the business failed, I'd have to apply to law school instead.

So, nearly a year after quitting alcohol, I started the Shamszad Group. I had only one client. I hustled for them until, next thing I knew, they referred a colleague. And then I had two. One client and one deal at a time, the business slowly but steadily grew. At least enough to save me from my dreaded law school contingency plan.

Chapter 5 - The Doctor Will See You, Again

You can't treat a mental illness while addicted to drugs or alcohol. Symptoms blur together. Episodes get accelerated. On any given day, I couldn't tell if I fought the illness or the addiction. Alcoholism and bipolar disorder are devastating in tandem. I used the former to mask the latter, all while treating neither.

But without alcohol, I could focus on the symptoms, triggers, and patterns of bipolar. I knew immediately that I wanted—needed—more control. I didn't want to be subject to the whims of the disorder, waiting for the next cycle of euphoria and despair. I faced a long, slow haul—one I'm still trudging.

I started by just taking my damn medicine on time, every day. In addition to the big, conspicuous, seven-day pill organizer I put in the bathroom, I put small stashes in my car, office, kitchen, and bathroom in case I forgot. Then I made—and kept—my appointments with the psychiatrist, Dr. Ewing. Part of me still resented him for locking the door on me. Even though I'd gone many months since my last drink and I'd formed a bit of perspective, I still didn't quite understand why he'd done it.

"Do you remember the last time I was here? When I was ten minutes late?"

"Of course, I do."

"I mean, I know I wasn't right on time, but why did you kick me out?"

"I understand how that must have felt, but—"

"Oh, do you?" I said, with a fraction of a smile.

"Let me finish. I understand how that must have felt, but that's a policy I have in place for a reason. My help is only as useful as my patients' own commitment to receiving it. The first step is showing up. And on time."

"But don't you think that can set someone back? I was in a bad place, man. I needed to see you. I needed help."

"If you needed to see me, why didn't you arrive on time?"

"I get it, but… I don't think it's that simple."

"Look, you are here, now. And I'm so glad to hear that you're sober. Keep it up. It's going to help you immensely. I hope I can be a part of your treatment."

I continued to see Dr. Ewing, and our meetings transformed from perfunctory prescription refills to deliberate treatment planning. He helped me understand bipolar disorder, fine-tuned my medication, and referred me to a therapist. She, in turn, re-introduced me to cognitive behavioral therapy, a practice I'd cursorily touched on while at Butler Hospital.

Equipping myself with an understanding of what bipolar disorder did to my mind helped me keep it at arm's length. I practiced recognizing specific thought patterns and steep mood vacillations for what they were—merely symptoms. And from there, I began to learn how to recognize the connection between my thoughts, moods, and subsequent behaviors. In that first year, I only scratched the surface of what would become an ongoing therapeutic undertaking. But it gave me a tool to chip away at the link between my thoughts and a reflexive desire to drink alcohol.

Unlike the endeavor to stop drinking, which I announced far and wide, my treatment for bipolar remained a private one. I talked to Will, Annie, and my mom, who was working towards her therapy license at the time. But my comfort stopped there—I had stretched my vulnerability to its capacity at the time. I didn't feel determined to *never* share it, but I wasn't ready. Not *yet*. I still had work to do. I needed to understand it and accept that it was an inextricable part of me, and that *that* was okay. In the meantime, I'd start the journey, one appointment at a time.

Chapter 6 - A Family Crest

On my first anniversary, I got a lot of texts, calls, and hugs. I answered questions about how I did it, what it felt like, and what was next. But I tried not to give way to too much celebration. I was scared to take my foot off the gas pedal and mistake a mile marker for a destination. Plus, it felt excruciating to rewind, replay, and relive what I'd done and where I'd been. It was, after all, the anniversary of one of the worst days of my life—waking up with blood all over me, nearly ready to die. A year later, it still felt like yesterday.

Around that time, a friend asked for some advice. I'd come to find it would be the first of many instances I'd serve as a confidant. He told me he'd been worried about his sister. She was in the throes of advanced alcoholism, without a partner or many friends to help. Her body and mind had become something he didn't recognize.

"When I picked her up at the airport, I wanted to be early, so I parked and waited for her inside. I thought I'd try to be at the baggage claim when she came down the escalator. When I saw her from a distance, she—"

He cut himself off and took a deep breath.

"It's all right, brother. Take your time." *It's okay, I understand. I was there.*

With his eyes closed, holding in tears, he said, "I wanted so bad for it to be someone else—you know, just some stranger that looked a bit like her from far away. But I knew it was her. Her head was sagging into her chest, and her legs were barely underneath her, man. There was a random lady with an arm around her, propping her up, making sure she didn't fall down the fucking stairs. She'd had so many damn drinks on the airplane that she couldn't even get to baggage claim."

At that moment, my head sank into my hands, and I started to weep. Minutes before, I was a pillar of empathy he could lean on for support. Then, before I knew it, I had fallen to pieces. Nothing but rubble where I had just stood tall. That's the power it still had—even a whole year later.

"I'm sorry, Dave. I didn't mean to stir all this up for you."

"No, no. It's okay. It's good. I just… I can see myself in her. And I can see you in all the people that were scared for me. But I am here for you. Both of you."

I'd come to learn that, in order to heal, it was essential to remember. To remain open to reflection and self-awareness. And perhaps to help others chart their paths. Addiction is a cold, dark place where the sun doesn't reach. It doesn't relent. It doesn't surrender. But we keep fighting. So that we never surrender, either. I'd grown strong enough to fight, scratch, and claw my way to the surface. But I knew the work would be unending. I had great days in that first year, where that nasty addiction appeared listless and bygone. Those days always passed and gave way to scared, frightful ones. But when they did, I stayed steeled and prepared, ready to fight and prevail.

So, to commemorate the first year, if not celebrate, I went to the grimy tattoo shop near our house and got a big, black phoenix on my shoulder. It roars at me every morning from its perch of ashes, rousing me for the day ahead. The blazing symbol of renewal is an homage to my dad, reminiscent of the silver pendant he donned all those years after he quit drinking. He and I now share a new family crest, celebrating the growth and evolution of our lineage. Generational trauma festers and compounds until it's exposed and countered through the steadfast resolve of brave guardians. Ones like my father, who declare, "No more. I will end this curse. For my children. And for theirs."

A few months before my second anniversary, I had one of the best days of my life. On a serendipitously sunny day, a chartered trolley car picked up my groomsmen—a weary but resilient troupe who'd stuck by my side—and me to take us to Shakespeare Garden in Golden Gate Park, where our friends and families awaited. My little sister, a brilliant musician, sang a beautiful love song. My widowed grandmother officiated.

My vows to her pledged a lifetime of companionship: "… I've needed support, and you've held me together during the worst of times… I now promise to be there for *you*. I vow to keep working to be a better partner, every day I'm alive."

Annie's vows spoke of an unyielding belief in one another: "… I promise to share my hopes and dreams with you, and look to you for strength and support… I give you this ring as a reminder of when our love was new, as it is now."

While my grandmother finished the ceremony, I leaned into that soft crevice between Annie's shoulder and her neck—the same place I longed to be when I woke up in Butler Hospital years and years ago. Just for her to hear, I whispered, "You saved my life. Thank you. I will always love you, forever, no matter what."

A couple of tears formed in her beautiful, sparkling green eyes. The smile she gave me at that moment… I will never forget it.

Chapter 7 - I Am Someone You Know

Years after I'd last seen him, Brandon, our brightest hope from the at-risk youth camp, sent me a message through Facebook. Annie and I had always believed Brandon could turn his life around if he wanted it badly enough. But he'd have obstacles to overcome—the stickiness of his juvenile record, the gravity of a former street life, and the elusiveness of second chances.

A chill ran through me when I saw his name. Was he just checking in on his old counselors? Could he be in trouble and in need of help? I then jumped to grave, even fearful, possibilities. What if this was a family member on his account letting his contacts know something bad had happened?

I had reason to feel uneasy. We'd recently learned that Juan had been murdered. He'd gone to prison for homicide and was stabbed to death inside. Ever since I saw Juan in the back seat of the police car, red and blue lights reflecting off his menacing grin, I'd wondered what more I could have done for him.

I let the message sit unread for about fifteen minutes, bracing myself for any possibility—the best, the worst, or, perhaps, simply spam sent from a hacked Facebook account.

Chief Dave? Is this you? It's Brandon from camp. Just wanted to say whatsup. I hope you're good, wherever you are. Lmk if you get this!

Yes! It's great to hear from you. I am doing good, thank you. Chief Annie and I are married and live in California. Would love to hear what you've been up to!

I'm great. I ended up finishing high school after I got out of camp. A few years after that, I actually went to culinary school. I'm a manager at a restaurant now and I am saving to open up my own place.

That's incredible! I'm so happy to hear that and I'm so proud of you. Annie and I haven't forgotten about you, of course. I can't wait to tell her.

I always think of you guys. I hope I see you again someday. You changed my life.

You changed my life. I read it over and over. A few tears cruised freely down my cheeks. I looked at his page. Joy overcame me when I saw the abstract of his life in pictures and stories. We had put our hearts into that place and those kids. All we ever wanted was to make some of their lives better. On the darkest days at camp, when we both wanted to run, we reminded ourselves that it would all be worthwhile if we could reach at least one.

It was an affirmation—a reminder that we all can change. It was not easy for Brandon. It was not easy for me. There's a gulf between the kinds of challenges we each faced. But both of us looked in the mirror and said, "No, I can fight. I *will* fight."

And that is the truth about courage. It's available to all of us, each and every day of our lives. We can find it at the crux of every obstacle. It's always there, waiting for us to grab hold of it. We are the authors of our own stories and it's never too late to write a new chapter. We don't often get to choose freedom from disease, affliction, mistakes made, or hardships endured. But we are always free to choose courage right *now*.

Millions of people fight addiction, mental illness, or both. Many suffer in the darkness and in silence, unseen and unheard. But they are right beside you. They are… someone you know.

Epilogue

A Proclamation

In that first year without alcohol, I began relearning what my body, mind, and heart could do. I'd been touched by the light of a new life, and I would not return to the shadows. But the recovery and healing were anything but perfunctory. The work was, and remains, unending.

I've now gone over a decade since that last drink. I have my health, a thriving business, and a loving family. Raw and overwhelming gratitude washes over me every day. Sometimes, I still don't believe it's real. I am living a dream—but one born of a nightmare. I'm lucky I survived. Lucky that Annie stayed with me. And luckier than ever to see her beautiful reflection in our little boy.

A few weeks into his first year of preschool, he came home especially jubilant, skipping around the house with long, sandy-blond hair flowing behind him. As usual, he rattled off the new words he'd picked up in class. But, on this day, instead of animals, shapes, and colors, he shouted, "I am me! I am me!"

At that, an unexpected exhilaration rushed through my body. His radiant smile, outstretched arms, and joyful confidence—my heart swelled, and my eyes bore a tear. He owned those words. His first decree of identity and self-belief. Oh, that we all could be so bold as to flash an untamed smile, reach up to the sky, and shout for all to hear, "I am me!"

Yes, baby boy, be you, indeed. Let your joy run wild whenever you see beauty around you. Be vulnerable with others and lead them with your heart. Give your strength when a friend needs it, but borrow theirs when yours is depleted. Be troubled and hurt. Be afflicted and suffer. But spurn the dubious notions of weakness and boldly ask for help. Set boundaries that make you safe, and shout "No!" when others tread over them. Be grateful for everything, but forgive yourself for wanting more. Make mistakes—lots of them—but let shame and guilt flow smoothly through you like water, and discover the opportunity to learn and grow.

Try out and miss the cut. But be relentless and go back for more. Stand up for someone and get a bloody nose. But also explore the power of forgiveness and empathy. Let the world know what you expect from it and do not relent when it won't yield to you. Wander outside the lanes you're assigned and give no regard to what others want you to be. Love who you love and tell them so. Howl at the moon from time to time. Or every damn night if it delights you. Cry when you need to and especially when you want to. Refrain when the time isn't right for the steep, arduous climbs. But, eventually, carry on, and do the hard things you know must be done.

With those daring, brash words, our two-year-old rocked the ground under my feet. I could see my whole life. A child, scared and alone. A teenager, fighting for another chance. And a young man, writhing in pain about to break under the weight of it. I could see the despair I'd suffered through and the love that I'd fought for. I could see... who I am.

I am a recovering alcoholic, one day away from another drink, if I falter. But a lifetime from one, too, if I choose courage. I am bipolar—

a cunning and maddening disorder. But I bless the virtues it has led me to—vulnerability and compassion.

I am our family's troubled child, forever adorned with the scars of our lineage. But I am our brilliant deliverance—with love for my own son extricated from an ancestral pain. I am an overjoyed father, brimming with excitement for every step he takes. But I am a frightened one, wary of my footsteps that he may follow. I am a devout partner—forever lovestruck and eternally grateful. But I am still learning to be selfless and truly one with another.

I am enterprising. Tenaciously building business and community. But I am novice, waking up every day with self-doubt and no-fucking-clue. I am fit, fast, and fierce—but only compared to the last iteration of myself. I am a phoenix rising from the despair of a former life. And yet, I am only just beginning—The fire rises still.

I am inspired by the brave ones that deal only in the truth, especially those that bare it all—despair, desire, loathing, and love. I am enraged by the bullies that feast on fear, particularly the biggest ones in the yard—our snarling, insidious voices of doubt.

I am thankful that I first picked up that bottle. I am glad to be vexed by this disorder. I do not regret the past. And I will not relent to shame. Every challenge and every obstacle led me to that beautiful moment… "I am me," you say? Yes, my love, goddamn fucking right you are.